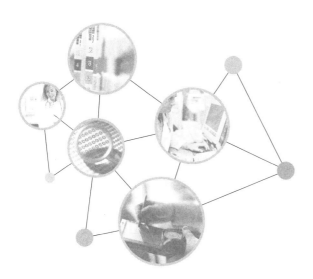

ELECTRONIC HEALTH RECORDS

Transforming Your Medical Practice

Margret Amatayakul
MBA, RHIA, CHPS, CPEHR, CPHIT, FHIMSS

Steven S. Lazarus
PhD, CPEHR, CPHIT, FHIMSS

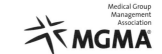

Medical Group
Management
Association

Medical Group Management Association
104 Inverness Terrace East
Englewood, CO 80112-5306
877.275.6462
Web site: www.mgma.com

Medical Group Management Association (MGMA) publications are intended to provide current and accurate information and are designed to assist readers in becoming more familiar with the subject matter covered. Such publications are distributed with the understanding that MGMA does not render any legal, accounting or other professional advice that may be construed as specifically applicable to individual situations. No representations or warranties are made concerning the application of legal or other principles discussed by the authors to any specific factual situation, nor is any prediction made concerning how any particular judge, government official, or other person will interpret or apply such principles. Specific factual situations should be discussed with professional advisors. MGMA neither represents nor endorses any particular company or commercial product or service mentioned by the authors or provided as explanation, examples or demonstration of the subject matter covered.

PUBLISHER'S CATALOGING-IN-PUBLICATION DATA

Amatayakul, Margret.
    Electronic health records: transforming your medical practice / Margret Amatayakul, Steven S. Lazarus.
    p. cm.
    Includes bibliographical references and index.
    ISBN 1-56829-232-5
    1. Medical records—Data processing. 2. Medical records—Management. 3. Medical offices—Data processing. 4. Information storage and retrieval systems—Medical care. 5. Medical offices—Management.
    I. Title: Electronic health records. II. Lazarus, Steven S. III. Title.
R864.A512 2005
610'.285—dc22
2005922617

Item #6266

Printed in the United States of America
10 9 8 7 6 5 4 3 2 1

CONTENTS 0101001011010010100101001000001000

LIST OF EXHIBITS   1101001010010100100001000

ABOUT THE AUTHORS 0101001010010000100

▶ **Margret Amatayakul**, MBA, RHIA, CHPS, CPEHR, CPHIT, FHIMSS, is president of Margret\A Consulting, LLC, a firm dedicated to providing effective and efficient solutions to today's information management and systems issues. She is also a co-founder of Health IT Certification.

Margret "A" has an extensive career history of working in the field of electronic health records and associated standards, such as the Health Insurance Portability and Accountability Act of 1996 (HIPAA). She has been director of health information management services at the Illinois Eye and Ear Infirmary, associate professor at the University of Illinois at the Medical Center, and associate executive director of the American Health Information Management Association (AHIMA). In addition, she helped found and was the first executive director of the Computer-based Patient Record Institute (CPRI), an organization that grew out of the recommendations in the first Institute of Medicine (IOM) patient record study (April 1991).

Margret is a widely acclaimed speaker and has published extensively, having several regular columns in health care trade magazines. She has written books on HIPAA, electronic health records, finance concepts for health professionals, and work flow and process improvement. Currently, she is also a clinical associate professor at the University of Illinois at Chicago and an adjunct faculty member in the master's in health informatics program at the College of St. Scholastica and on its ATHENS Project advisory committee. This committee, in partnership with a major health information services vendor, focuses on integrating computer-based clinical information system applications into health sciences professional curricula.

Margret is a registered health information administrator (RHIA); is certified in healthcare privacy and security (CHPS), electronic health records (CPEHR), and health information technology (CPHIT); and is a Fellow of the Healthcare Information and Management Systems Society (FHIMSS). She is also serving on the HIMSS board of directors and is on the certification process work group of the Certification Commission for Healthcare

Information Technology. She has also served as a contractor to the National Committee on Vital and Health Statistics (NCVHS) on its patient medical record information and electronic prescribing (e-prescribing) standards recommendations. She has a bachelor's degree in medical record administration from the University of Illinois at the Medical Center and a master's degree in business administration with concentrations in marketing and finance from the University of Illinois at Chicago.

▶ **Steven S. Lazarus**, PhD, CPEHR, CPHIT, FHIMSS, is president and co-founder of Boundary Information Group (BIG), a consortium of health care information and technology consulting firms using their collective experience and knowledge to address the information needs of the health care community. He consults on electronic health records, system strategic planning, revenue cycle and work flow improvement, and HIPAA compliance. His clients include physician practices, hospitals, insurance companies, vendors, government (federal, state and local), and national associations.

Steve currently serves on the Workgroup for Electronic Data Interchange (WEDI) board of directors (he is the past chair of the board) and is a WEDI Foundation Trustee. From 1990 to 1994, he was an executive responsible for research and information systems activities at the Medical Group Management Association (MGMA).

In 2004, Steve co-founded Health IT Certification, LLC, an electronic health record and health information technology professional training and certification program. At the National HIPAA Summit on October 31, 2002, Steve received the Extraordinary Achievement Award for his contribution to the health care community by facilitating the development and implementation of the HIPAA law and regulations. He also is the recipient of WEDI's 2002 Vision and Leadership Award as WEDI chairman.

Steve received a bachelor's degree in industrial engineering from Cornell University and a master's degree in industrial engineering and operations research from Polytechnic University. The University of Rochester awarded him a doctorate in business administration. He is a certified professional in electronic health records (CPEHR) and health information technology (CPHIT), and is a Fellow of the Healthcare Information and Management Systems Society (FHIMSS).

Today's level of interest in electronic health records (EHRs) has been spawned by many factors – not the least of which is gaining recognition for the role information technology plays in our everyday society. Being mindful of EHRs has many facets. Just as medical practices evaluate any major capital expenditure, they need to consider not only the financial investment but the degree of change for which they are ready. Changes brought about by an EHR should result in improvements, and the opportunities need to be understood and anticipated. The purpose of this book, then, is to introduce all aspects of EHR definition, planning, vendor selection, acquisition, implementation, adoption, and benefits realization.

EHRs are on the minds of almost every physician in practice today. For those who recognize an EHR will need to be their next capital investment, there is very likely much to learn and consider; at a minimum, tips from those who have gone before are always helpful. There may also be many practices that need to better understand the full scope of what an EHR means, how to approach adoption of information technology in a meaningful way, and what traps should be avoided. Even those whose practice has acquired an EHR may be considering the next enhancement or determining how to optimize its use.

From soup to nuts, this book goes from introducing you to EHRs and providing a rationale for EHR acquisition to offering a case study that illustrates success achieved and lessons learned.

CHAPTER 1 – Introduction and Rationale for EHRs describes the EHR, offering terms and definitions often associated with EHR and other information technology. It discusses the strategic options for an EHR and various components of a comprehensive EHR system. It highlights the benefits of EHR implementation and helps you to recognize the types of changes in operations and work flow needed to achieve those benefits. Finally, this chapter helps you anticipate potential barriers and offers suggestions for ways to overcome them.

CHAPTER 2 – EHR Technology is essentially a technical primer for those who want or need a more thorough understanding of the basic computer technology that supports an EHR. It describes hardware components of EHRs including special attention on human-computer interfaces, networking and communication requirements, the various operating system platforms on which EHRs are built, and the types of application software that make up an EHR. This chapter helps you to appreciate the standards you should look for in an EHR to ensure interoperability and data comparability and to understand how data are managed within a database. It also address security measures in general to protect confidentiality, ensure data integrity, and support continual availability to your data.

CHAPTER 3 – Determining Your Group's Objectives helps you to determine your group's objectives for the EHR. It describes various levels of benefits that may be achieved based on the level of EHR sophistication to be acquired. This chapter also offers considerations that should be made based on the size and specialty of the group. Organizing this information can help you plot a migration path from your current position to where you plan to be in the future with an EHR.

CHAPTER 4 – Return on Investment addresses the critical issue of return on investment (ROI). It helps you quantify benefits from EHR systems, identify and develop financial benefits assumptions, identify costs of EHR systems, calculate ROI payback period for an EHR system, and understand other ROI measures. This chapter gives you an appreciation of the value of a benefits realization activity.

CHAPTER 5 – Determining and Managing Your Requirements is designed to prepare you to go to market for an EHR. It describes the relationships among the EHR, practice management and/or billing system(s), and other information system applications. Most important, it helps you to identify and describe the features and functions an EHR must have to support your projected benefits and to determine any special considerations that need to be addressed. Special considerations include those from the perspective of your specialty, hospital/practice relationships, communications with other providers/patients, or those for compliance with accreditation, licensure, or other legal and regulatory requirements. This chapter also helps you to learn how an EHR may require work flow redesign and process improvements, and potentially even layout and furnishing changes to achieve your projected benefits.

CHAPTER 6 – How to Select the Right Vendor and EHR for Your Practice outlines a series of steps to take as you select the right EHR for your practice. It helps you to understand the process of identifying your requirements and matching them to the product offerings of the EHR vendor community. This chapter also describes how to construct an EHR implementation and ongoing operations budget. It describes in detail the important step of preparing a request for proposal and the process to utilize this document effectively in your vendor selection process. This chapter includes data gathering and review processes to help you to review your requirements on a phased basis and choose the vendor EHR products most closely matching your current and future needs.

CHAPTER 7 – Planning and Initiating an EHR Implementation discusses EHR implementation through final testing. It guides you through a process based on a structured project plan. It includes a discussion on the importance of both your organization and your vendor assigning resources, including personnel, to the implementation based on your plan. The discussion also guides you to monitor and address budget, technical, and testing issues as they occur during implementation. This chapter helps you to learn how to determine the work flow customization for your practice to assess the alternatives for converting paper medical charts into the EHR at the time you "go live."

CHAPTER 8 – Implementation and Ongoing Operations helps you to understand how to manage the implementation and ongoing operations of your EHR. It shows how to phase-in the EHR implementation and manage the conversion of paper records. This chapter discusses the importance of and resources needed to deploy training and support for the initial implementation as well as on an ongoing basis to assure that your EHR is maintained and kept current with future enhancements offered by your vendor. It emphasizes the importance of managing unexpected challenges and problems that will arise during EHR implementation and ongoing maintenance, as well as how to work collaboratively with your vendor and manage the vendor payment process based on successful implementation.

CHAPTER 9 – The EHR Regulatory and Standards Environment provides a comprehensive description of resources available to you relating to data standards, transaction standards, and the interoperability of sharing health care data within and among organizations. It shows you how to monitor the relevant sources of information available from the federal government, standards developing organizations (SDOs), and other sources, and how to identify the more important types of information available from an EHR perspective.

CHAPTER 10 – EHR Case Study presents a case study that describes the experience of a medical group going through the process of planning for, selecting, and implementing an EHR. It includes examples that contributed significantly to a successful implementation and illustrates the types of issues that you might encounter in this complex process.

▼ ▼ ▼

This book specifically focuses on the individuals who need to help medical group practices make the best decisions concerning information technology investment. However, anyone needing to understand EHRs will benefit from reading this book:

▶ For practice administrators, the book offers step-by-step guidance on understanding the practice's readiness for an EHR, how to plan a migration path to achieve the most benefits, and specifically how to set up and manage an EHR selection and implementation process.

▶ For physicians and other clinicians in the practice, the book describes the scope and impact an EHR will have on how to perform day-to-day activities. It helps debunk myths, overcome misperceptions, and ensure an understanding of the realities.

▶ For board members who may want a more thorough understanding of what the EHR investment entails, the book describes what others have accomplished through EHRs, what pitfalls need to be addressed, and how to establish appropriate expectations for return on investment.

▶ For information systems support personnel or contractors who may not have experience with implementing clinical systems, the book provides a primer on clinical practice and how that is impacted by the EHR.

In summary, this book emphasizes the clinical transformation that an EHR achieves. An EHR is not merely a software application that helps in managing a practice. It is a system of hardware, software, people, policy, and process that helps to improve the effectiveness and efficiency of health care.

ACKNOWLEDGMENTS 0100101001000010011

Throughout our careers, it has been our good fortune to have worked with so many knowledgeable and encouraging professionals, who, like most in the medical field, are deeply committed to providing quality health care. Many with whom we have worked as clients, management consulting colleagues, and professional association collaborators have provided us the opportunity to share our ideas and expertise for improving the delivery of health care through the use of electronic health records and information systems.

For five years, Steve Lazarus was the executive manager responsible for the Center for Research in Ambulatory Health Care Administration (CRAHCA), an affiliate organization of the Medical Group Management Association (MGMA). Collaborations with MGMA staff, leadership, and members during those years and since then are very much appreciated. Several of the projects that were undertaken during his tenure at MGMA have contributed to the conceptual development of the use of electronic health records in medical groups.

We want to thank our MGMA colleagues, who contributed to the direction and stimulated our approach to this book. Our grateful appreciation especially goes to three individuals who have been particularly helpful throughout this process: Marti Cox, information resources manager; Carolyn Lyons, director, Information Center and Knowledge Management; and Robert Tennant, senior policy advisor. In addition, we want to thank Sandra Rush for her editing skills and recommendations, and Jean Van Horn, administrative assistant at Boundary Information Group, for her excellent help in the production of this book.

We would also like to acknowledge our families, who encouraged our writing of this book and have continuously been supportive of our work in the health care industry.

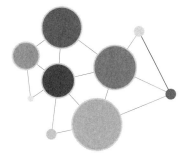

 ONE

Introduction and Rationale for EHRs

Using the power of computers is now common in many physician practices. Computers are now being used for a wide range of applications. Billing is usually the first application to be automated. A practice management system (PMS) offers additional help with scheduling, registration, and chart tracking. Many physician practices connect electronically to hospitals and laboratories for access to results and other clinical messaging services. Electronic prescribing (e-prescribing) tools are also becoming popular.

Many initiatives point to the fact that this is the era of the electronic health record. The federal government is promoting the use of health information technology (HIT) for patient safety and enhanced quality of care. Payers have started pay-for-performance (P4P) efforts that virtually require an EHR for physicians to meet data reporting needs. In addition, local and regional information infrastructures are being formed.

THIS CHAPTER PROVIDES an introduction and presents rationale for physician group practices to take the next major step in computerization. Specifically, the chapter helps you:

 Understand the evolution of EHRs, including associated terms;

 Appreciate the strategic options for an EHR and the components it comprises;

 Identify the potential benefits of an EHR;

▶ Recognize changes in operations and work flow needed for a successful EHR implementation;

▶ Recognize ways to overcome potential barriers to an EHR; and

▶ Plan the overall process of selecting and implementing an EHR.

▶ Evolution of EHRs

The first commercially used computers came about in the mid-1950s, with their ability to "crunch" large amounts of numbers tirelessly and accurately (as long as the machines were programmed correctly). Businesses adopted computers to perform various accounting and other financial applications.

The first use of computers in health care occurred in the mid-1960s.[1] The initial belief was that computers could aid in managing the operations of provider organizations and help document patient conditions. This was a much bigger challenge, however, than merely performing bookkeeping or inventory functions. As a result, the first processes to be automated were similar to those in other industries, such as billing and patient accounting, the generation of work lists for laboratory specimen collection, and inventory management in the pharmacy. Some time later, more complex health care processes began to be successfully addressed.

The increasing complexity of the reimbursement process also contributed to the use of computers for abstracting data from medical records to apply to claims and ultimately to manage reimbursement contracting. The Uniform Hospital Discharge Data Set (UHDDS), the basis of hospital discharge data systems in many states, was developed in 1985. Subsequently other data sets have been adopted for reporting data in long-term care, home health care, and other types of health care facilities. The International Classification of Diseases (ICD), which was originally developed solely to classify causes of mortality and morbidity for research and public health purposes, has also been enhanced for use in coding diagnoses, and in coding procedures for hospital reimbursement purposes. The American Medical Association produced the Current Procedural Terminology (CPT®) code system, not only to help establish billing rates but also to help automate the billing process. These were adopted under the Health Insurance Portability and Accountability Act of 1996 (HIPAA) for use in electronic claims processing as well. Many experts today believe similar data sets may be required for physician practices, especially as a P4P model is introduced by payers.[2]

As technology improved over the years, so did the computer applications that were available to health care organizations. Physician practices became interested in automating more than just accounting functions. Many physician practices investigated the automation of appointment scheduling systems, registration systems, master patient indexes, and other practice management functions. The result was the development of PMSs that integrate many of these operational and financial applications into one system.

Automating the entire content of the medical record and associated processes, however, presents challenges. Even though handwritten documents can be scanned into a computer and retrieved for later review, such a system does not lend itself to collecting data for data sets and certainly not to supporting other processes. Such a system can't "read" entries in a chart at the time they are made, for example, and offer suggestions for missing data needed for reimbursement coding. It cannot compare, in real time, the drugs being considered for a patient against a payer's formulary to determine their cost, nor recognize that there may be contraindications with other drugs the patient is taking.

Classification systems such as ICD or CPT may be suitable for public health and reimbursement, but they do not provide sufficient detail for processing the data used to make diagnosis and treatment decisions. To fully automate the medical record, each term used to describe a patient's medical history, symptoms, physical findings, test results, and so forth, must be encoded by the computer. Computer processing of medical terms depends on a precise meaning being associated with each term as well as the computer "understanding" relationships between terms. The College of American Pathologists (CAP) has been working since the early 1970s to develop a clinical language standard of medicine that could be used to encode medical terms and their relationships for use in computers. The resultant Systematized Nomenclature of Medicine, Clinical Terms (SNOMED CT®) is now becoming an international standard for computer encoding of medical terms. Likewise, laboratory and other diagnostic study results are being encoded by a system developed and maintained by the Regenstrief Institute, namely, Logical Observation Identifiers Names and Codes® (LOINC®).

Today, with more sophisticated computer technology, we are learning how to develop highly complex processing structures that can manage huge amounts of information from multiple sources and present the right information at the point of care. Privacy and security, legislated through HIPAA,[3] are incorporated into information systems to ensure timely access to information for appropriately authorized individuals and safe utilization of the transmission capabilities of the Internet.[4]

▶ EHR Terminology

As a result of the evolution toward more robust computers providing more effective and efficient capture and use of health information, the terms that have come to be associated with EHRs are many and varied. Exhibit 1.1 provides a listing and definitions of some of the most commonly used terms. Some experts view differences in terms as an evolutionary process of increasing sophistication.[5] Others believe different terms are generally synonymous, often reflecting vendors' different interpretations or their desire to distinguish their products.[6] In some cases, different terms are used to describe components of, or adjuncts to, EHR systems. Some terms are more popular for physician practice systems; others are more commonly used for hospital or long-term care systems.

EXHIBIT 1.1   EHR Terms   1010010110100101001010010000010001100

Electronic health record (EHR) – This term is currently used to describe the broadest scope of health information computing. EHR has been legitimized by the Health Level Seven® (HL7®) standards group, which has recently provided the first "official" definition of EHR functionality.[7]

Electronic medical record (EMR) – This term has been the one most commonly used for EHRs in physician practices. When used in reference to hospital information systems, it may suggest only a document imaging version of an EHR.

Computer-based patient record (CPR) – Generally considered synonymous with EHR, this term was coined by the Institute of Medicine in its 1991 landmark report, *The Computer-based Patient Record: An Essential Technology for Healthcare*.[8] This report suggested for the first time that EHR was more than just an automated version of the paper record – it was a longitudinal record of patient care with enhanced utility beyond documentary evidence of care rendered.

Electronic patient record (EPR) – This term may have been coined because "CPR" also stands for cardiopulmonary resuscitation. Some experts suggest it is similar to the computer-based patient record, but not as inclusive.

EXHIBIT 1.1 EHR Terms *continued* 0110100101001010010000010001100

Automated medical record (AMR) – This term was used early in the evolution of EHRs to convey the notion of automating processes associated with medical record documentation; the term is rarely used today.

Computerized medical record (CMR) – This term is sometimes used to describe a document imaging system, which tends to be considered a precursor, or bridge, to a full EHR.

Digital medical record (DMR) – This term is sometimes used to describe a Web-based patient record using "pull" technology. This type of system is more frequently referred to as a clinical messaging system, by which results can be retrieved from a remote source.

Patient medical record information (PMRI) – This term was used in the HIPAA Administrative Simplification provisions, which required the National Committee on Vital and Health Statistics (NCVHS) to make recommendations for uniform data standards for the electronic exchange of patient medical record information.[9] The intent of the use of this term was to promote standards development and adoption without requiring the implementation of a specific system.

Personal health record (PHR) – This is a relatively new concept wherein the patient or other caregiver compiles information from a variety of providers as well as self-reported information.[10] The PHR has a variety of forms, from records maintained by providers, often through a Web portal to fax-back services that provide clearinghouse functions for patient information; to records maintained solely by the patient, either electronically or on paper. The PHR may also be called a patient-carried record (PCR).

Continuity of care record (CCR) – This is a new concept that has emerged from the American Academy of Family Practice, American Academy of Pediatrics, the Massachusetts Medical Society and other groups, in concert with the standards development organization ASTM International.[11] This is primarily a standard set of data that would be exchanged between referring physicians.

Integrated care record services (ICRS) – This term is primarily used in the United Kingdom to describe functionality somewhat similar to the CCR.

Computerized health information systems (CHIS) – This is a generic term used to describe the set of health information applications that are computerized, often in a hospital. The totality of the CHIS may lead to the ability to more effectively implement an EHR.

EXHIBIT 1.1   EHR Terms *continued*   0110100101001010010000010001100

Patient care record (PCR) – This is the term most often used to reflect computerization of nursing and other clinical documentation in a hospital. It is different from a patient-carried, or personal health, record (PHR).

Computerized provider order entry (CPOE) – This is a system that captures and routes orders. A CPOE system supports the capture of complete and accurate order information entered directly by the provider authorized to write orders, and it also offers clinical decision support that provides alerts and reminders concerning contraindications, appropriate dosing, duplicate procedures, in-formulary advice, and so forth. Although primarily used in hospitals, CPOE may be used in large medical groups that have in-house laboratories, physical therapists and other services. This differs from order communication systems, in which clerical personnel transcribe a provider's handwritten orders for transmission.

Electronic prescribing (e-prescribing) – This is a system that computerizes the writing of prescriptions and their transmission to retail pharmacies. It may be as simple as an up-to-date formulary on a handheld device to a system supported by an EHR that provides for the capture of a complete prescription with clinical decision support.[12] Although e-prescribing systems are primarily used by providers in group practices or physician practices, they may also be used to write hospital discharge orders for medication prescriptions that will be filled at a retail pharmacy and for prescription writing in hospital outpatient departments and clinics.

Clinical decision support system (CDSS) – This is a component of an EHR that provides alerts, reminders, access to knowledge sources (such as medical literature, research studies, and drug knowledge bases), structured data entry tools to ensure complete and accurate recording of information, and other aids that help providers manage quality of care and attend to patient safety issues.[13]

Clinical data repository (CDR) – This is a component of an EHR that receives data from multiple sources and stores it for online, real-time access to the data. A clinical data warehouse (CDW) is a set of data that may be derived from a data repository and is generally used to process retrospective analyses on data.

▶ What is an EHR?

As suggested in Exhibit 1.1, the term "electronic health record" is the currently used term to describe the fullest degree of functionality in health information computing. It has become the standard term most widely used in health care today. Differences in what vendors sell as "EHR systems" may still be significant, and there certainly can be a migration path from simple to sophisticated. However, understanding with respect to the ultimate vision of the EHR is coming together, and most experts today agree that the concepts provided in Exhibit 1.2 define an EHR.

EXHIBIT 1.2 EHR Definition 100101101001010010100100001000011100

An EHR is a system (of hardware, software, people, policies, and processes) that:

▶ Collects data from multiple sources;

▶ Is used by clinicians as the primary source of information at the point of care; and

▶ Provides decision support for evidence-based health care.

System

When an EHR is described as a "system," it means that hardware, software, people, policies, and processes work together to collect data and provide information and decision support (e.g., alerts, reminders) to the clinician (and other users as applicable) whenever and wherever the information is needed.

An EHR system typically builds upon computer systems that are already in place for billing and/or practice management. If your practice does not have such a system, you might consider an EHR that includes PMS functions, or implement a PMS before implementing an EHR.

Hardware

Hardware refers to the computer and network equipment on which applications run. This equipment includes devices that provide the ability for persons to enter data into the computer, sometimes referred to as human-computer interfaces (HCIs).

Software

Software refers to the instructional programs developed to make computers work. The programs you license from a vendor to use in your practice, such as a billing system, PMS, or EHR are examples of application software. Some of these, such as the EHR, are very sophisticated and include special types of databases. As you enter data into the EHR, the data are going into a clinical data repository (CDR). Some databases contain branching logic that supports the EHR's alerting and reminder system. These databases are sometimes called rules engines and are used for clinical decision support systems (CDSS). Databases may also provide special information that comes from subscription services, or knowledge sources. For example, you may subscribe to a drug formulary service that periodically provides updated information about new drugs. Sometimes the EHR collects so much information that selected data are copied into a clinical data warehouse (CDW) for special analytical processing.

People

Probably the most critical elements in the EHR system are the people. When physician practices start thinking about acquiring the hardware and software for an EHR system, they sometimes pay more attention to the devices than to the people, policies, and processes that must make the system work. It is always important to recognize that some of the people expected to use the system might not be regular computer users and therefore might need special assistance in learning computer basics. All of the people expected to use the system will need training on the special applications that make up an EHR system.

Many practices are also providing information to their patients about what their EHRs can do for them. Some EHR vendors put up "under construction" signs to alert patients that a practice is undergoing EHR implementation that may temporarily slow down registration or alter other processes. Many providers have made it a point to describe to their patients how they plan to use the EHR, how it will benefit them, and, if applicable, how they may interact with it via e-mail or gain access to their personal health records (PHRs) through a patient portal (a secure entry point from the Internet to a practice's Web page).

Providers increasingly are wanting to share data with other providers. They may need to send data for a patient referral or supply a continuity of care record (CCR) to another provider who is taking over the patient's care. Providers who need to access data from the hospital, lab, nursing home, or other facility where they practice can use a provider portal for this purpose.

Policies

Policies for use help to direct not only how the systems will generally be used but also the specific nature of how the applications process data. For example, if a practice wants to accept e-mail from patients, it should have a policy that describes how that will be performed to ensure it is used appropriately (e.g., not for emergencies) and in a confidential and secure manner. Policies also direct specifically how the EHR will work. For example, a practice may have a policy that requires providers to always check a drug formulary before prescribing certain types of drugs. This policy will be translated into the computer programs in the form of an alert when a provider attempts to write a prescription for such a drug and hasn't checked the formulary, or the computer can automatically check the formulary before confirming that the prescription is ready for signature or alerting that it needs to be revised based on formulary information.

Processes

Processes are the ways people perform work. Computer systems change the way people apply policies, resulting in changing processes. Although it is important not to disrupt clinical processes that ensure quality of care and patient safety, many EHR systems can automate components of these processes to enhance their results. EHR systems should result in changes that improve productivity in the practice so there is more time to take care of patients. For example, eliminating the volume of calls from pharmacies relating to unreadable prescriptions, prescriptions for off-formulary medications, or prescription contraindications identified by the pharmacist has been found to save considerable time for both the provider and the patient. In addition, the filing of paper charts should be greatly reduced or even eliminated through EHR implementation. Staff time previously used to perform these functions may be used to scan documents from external sources or documents (such as consent forms) that must be signed by the patient. Staff may be used to perform new customer service functions, such as calling patients on a list the computer has generated to remind them of the need for a checkup. If there is a patient portal component to the EHR that provides for patient access to lab results or provides patients the ability to schedule appointments or send e-mail to providers, staff who previously filed charts may be used to manage some of the incoming and outgoing messages or to keep the Web site up to date.

An EHR, then, is truly a *system* of devices, programs, users, support mechanisms and improvements that help not only to document care, but, properly implemented, to improve the provision of care. Exhibit 1.3 is a schematic drawing of the application components that are generally considered necessary to perform the full range of functions of an EHR. Keep in mind, however, that many providers start with clinical messaging, document imaging or a documentation system that is not as comprehensive as that illustrated in Exhibit 1.3.

EXHIBIT 1.3 EHR Components 1011010010101001010010000010001100

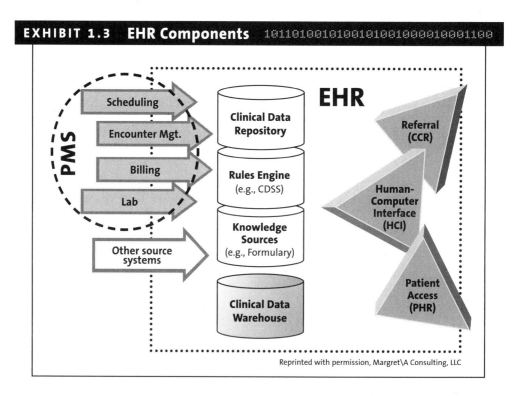

Reprinted with permission, Margret\A Consulting, LLC

▶ Achieving EHR Benefits

Despite advances in medical technology, the health care industry lags behind other industries in adopting technology to process its information. Even when a practice has automated its billing functions or added a PMS to help manage its operations, the core data that clinicians rely on to treat patients is still primarily embedded in paper files that often are difficult to locate, cannot be used simultaneously by more than one person, are possibly illegible, or may even be incomplete.

In addition, paper charts do not perform work. They cannot issue an alert when new lab results arrive, indicate when a result is critical, or track those results over time for a patient. Paper files often create more work due to their inadequacies. Managing refill requests can be a nightmare of telephone tag and post-it notes that are misplaced. Documenting medical necessity can be a puzzle often not solved, resulting in lower revenue. Lack of reminders for health maintenance checks can result in missed opportunities for improving patient care as well as lack of evidence for managed care contracting. As a result of these and many other issues, staff who depend on paper files must constantly create lab logs, refill folders, check formulary notebooks, duplicate encounter forms, and perform many other tedious functions.

Just as a solid billing system has helped improve back-office functions and a PMS has helped improve front-office functions, an EHR helps improve the core function of health care – in the examining room and beyond. Although the benefits to be achieved by an EHR are powerful, they may also be more subtle, however, and may take a long time and much effort to achieve. This difference is primarily because an EHR often is phased in and requires thoughtful "system building" and careful adjustments to processes over time. For example, a practice may be uncomfortable with "going paperless" immediately upon implementing an EHR, and it may take a year or more before clinicians are comfortable relying totally on the EHR for patient data. It may also take this long to transition information from current paper charts to the EHR.

Benefits from EHR systems may be characterized in a variety of ways. Some benefits are easier to quantify than others:

> ▶ *Quantifiable benefits* are those that can be described specifically by cost savings, revenue increases, percent change, time differences, or other numeric values. For example, paperless charts can help a practice reduce or even eliminate transcription costs. Decision support for coding can help increase revenues. The number of missed appointments may be reduced, or scores on a patient satisfaction survey may be increased. Clinicians may find they can go home earlier (or see more patients) on most days because they don't have to spend time to complete charts.

▶ *Anecdotal benefits* are benefits that cannot easily be quantified. They are no less important than quantifiable benefits, and in some cases they are more important. They often are described by specific case studies. For example, a clinician may recall that an allergy warning coupled with access to an online drug knowledge source helped identify the most appropriate drug for Mrs. Jones. Or, having Mr. Smith's X-rays available online to compare over time helped a physician recognize a problem before it became too severe.

Benefits may also be described as they relate to monetary value or quality:

▶ *Financial benefits* are those that have monetary value. Most EHR systems require a fairly significant financial investment, and practices want to be able to understand their return on investment (ROI). Anticipating financial benefits is important in making a decision about the affordability of the system. Chapter 4 is devoted to determining ROI.

▶ *Qualitative benefits* are also important, even though they do not directly contribute to "paying" for the system. Qualitative benefits accrue to clinicians, the practice itself, patients, and the general health status of the population. They may be as simple as reducing the hassle factor. Always having a chart available when needed is a huge improvement for practice morale and clinician satisfaction. Reducing the number of calls and increasing the time available to care for patients is a definite plus for clinicians.

Qualitative benefits of an EHR include knowing you are improving the quality of care in your practice. Many patient safety benefits are qualitative. The reduction in medication errors is often cited as a key benefit because an EHR can provide drug-drug, drug-lab, or drug-allergy alerts. Improved compliance with a treatment regimen may result from instructions generated from the EHR that are tailored specifically to the patient. Instantaneous access to medical literature may help in differential diagnosis and faster or more specific treatment for unusual cases. With the increasing emphasis on privacy and confidentiality, EHR can support information security efforts. Qualitative benefits may include a reduction in the spread of communicable disease through more complete and timely public health reporting, or even recognition of a potential bioterrorism threat. Drug or device recalls can be managed easily with a query to the computer system, automatic generation of notices, and potentially even auto-dial telephony capability.

Perhaps the most important factor in understanding the potential benefits of an EHR is to recognize that there is a benefits portfolio – comprising many different types of benefits. Paying for the system is critical, but other benefits can be very satisfying and important. Many anecdotal and qualitative benefits lead to downstream financial benefits, but are just more difficult to quantify.

Another important factor to bear in mind when analyzing benefits is to recognize that practices vary greatly. Vendors and others can provide guidance on the types of benefits that can be realized, but only those in the practice really know how the EHR can work in their particular environment.

▶ Managing Change in Operations and Work Flow

In fact, knowing the practice is a critical element in achieving anticipated benefits from an EHR. This means that selecting the right EHR at the right time requires the right reasons. The reasons come from truly understanding the practice – its culture, its values, its strengths and weaknesses, and its adaptability to change.

Change Management

Some vendors tout EHR systems that "don't change your practice." Spending a significant amount of time and money to have nothing change doesn't seem right, just as change for the sake of change is clearly wrong. Changes to achieve the benefits cited thus far will impact operations and work flow in the practice. If you have implemented a billing system and/or a PMS, you may have already introduced some operational changes. Having clinicians use the EHR for all aspects of their work, however, is generally a much bigger change than that brought about by a billing system or PMS. Some of these changes have already been suggested. Others will depend on the system you select and will be discussed further in subsequent chapters. Even some apparently simple changes, such as repositioning furniture in the examining rooms for the most effective use of the EHR, can take on significant importance.

Some groups are more than ready to take on an EHR and the changes in operations and work flow that result – they know their current policies and processes need updating and improvement. Other practices may already be fairly streamlined and want to enhance that capability further. For them, change has probably been a way of life over time. Yet other practices may recognize the need for some changes but face some reluctance to give up old ways or may have other forms of resistance to overcome.

Migration Path

The degree of change can be mitigated to a certain extent by starting with a less sophisticated system and phasing in various modifications. For example, if the practice knows it will take several years to convince clinicians to use a computer directly, it may be appropriate to start with a document imaging system. At least the benefits of record availability can be achieved. Another approach is to institute clinical messaging, especially where communication across multiple providers and/or multiple settings poses a challenge. If the practice is large enough, it may be appropriate to implement an EHR in one location or with one group of physicians to "work out the kinks." However, the practice should be aware that sometimes a phased-in approach only makes the pain of change last longer, developing more resistance as it goes along. In addition, this generally means running parallel processes (one for the paper-based system and another for the EHR) or having a hybrid record system in which part is on paper and part is in a computer. This situation can generate more work and more errors if not carefully managed.

Leadership

Change management is an important skill to bring to an EHR project. But as with predicting benefits, apply caution in how change management is performed. Many change management tools and techniques exist – some can be helpful, but some introduce bureaucracy and even greater resistance to change.

Some key principles in effecting change are basic leadership and team building. The clinicians in the practice will be the primary users of an EHR, but everyone in the practice is impacted in some way. Whether the practice's formal leadership directs the EHR initiative or appoints a project manager, all persons in the practice absolutely must have some involvement in EHR visioning, migration path development, selection, implementation, and adoption. In fact, valuing each practice member's role in EHR adoption is probably the most critical step in achieving its benefits.

Exhibit 1.4 identifies some of the qualifications and skills a person being considered for project manager should have. Note that an information technology (IT) background is not required, as consultants or the vendor

EXHIBIT 1.4   EHR Project Manager Qualifications and Skills 100

An EHR project manager should be able to:

1. Become familiar with the EHR system's functionality, technology, costs, and benefits;

2. Conduct an operations and work flow analysis to identify potential functions for the EHR:

   a. Conduct an inventory of existing information systems to ensure they can connect with the EHR (for practices with multiple systems);

   b. Trace the flow of processes that will be impacted by the EHR to understand how they are currently performed and what changes may be applicable for an EHR;

   c. Measure the volume and/or time it takes to perform these processes, if desired, to conduct a cost-benefit analysis and/or benefits realization study;

3. Review vendor offerings and make recommendations for review of those most suitable for the practice;

4. Develop a request for proposal (RFP), manage receipt of responses, analyze results, and present findings; in addition, arrange for demonstrations as applicable;

5. Manage the vendor selection process to ensure a fair analysis and unbiased selection; utilize information systems and financial and legal consultants as may be necessary to help in narrowing the field: calculate ROI and arrange financing for the project, and negotiate a contract;

6. Lead the internal implementation team – depending on the size of the practice and complexity of the EHR system, this may entail installation, system building and training, or coordinating vendor implementation activities;

7. Monitor adoption and use routinely and take corrective action as necessary; and

8. Apply updates as applicable, evaluate and recommend upgrades and enhancements, and work with users to develop reports and other uses of EHR data.

An EHR project manager should have the following knowledge and skills:

1. Familiarity with the health care practice or other similar health care practices;

2. A general understanding of computers and appreciation for information systems theory and design;

3. Analytical skills to identify problems and offer solutions;

4. Political and people skills to effectively manage change; and

5. Business acumen and insight into clinical processes.

Reprinted with permission, Margret\A Consulting, LLC

may generally fill this role. A clinical background is not necessarily an essential prerequisite either, as the practice team should provide that knowledge base.

▶ Overcoming Barriers to EHRs

Many group practices may believe that the single greatest barrier to obtaining an EHR is cost. Although cost is certainly a substantial consideration, often the greatest barrier is overcoming resistance to the change processes described in the preceding section.

Cost

The cost of EHR hardware and software – whether those are purchased, licensed or leased – can be substantial. Costs also vary widely between systems and applications. To gain a good understanding of the actual costs, it is important to fully understand the technology available and then determine your group's specific objectives. Some experts estimate that the cost of an EHR can be between $25,000 and $50,000 per provider in the practice. Some systems that can contribute to focused improvements can cost less, and other systems can be extremely comprehensive and cost more. Payback periods for EHR systems generally range from 2 to 5 years. Achieving an ROI, again, depends on the scope of functionality acquired, rate of adoption, and the level of incremental change in processes.

In addition to direct costs are the indirect costs of learning the system, customizing it to meet your practice's needs, adapting processes to achieve the benefits of the EHR, and maintaining the system. Some practices find it best to reduce patient load for a few weeks during the "go live" period, and this cost must be factored into the total expense. Many practices also find it essential that one or more clinicians serve as champions and spend considerable time helping in the vendor selection, developing tailored templates and reports, implementing clinical guidelines, training others, and monitoring the environment for enhancements. Many practices negotiate compensation for these clinicians or, in larger practices, promote them to informatics positions, replacing at least some of their clinical time.

Other Barriers

Other barriers that have been identified when practices think about acquiring EHRs include legal, regulatory, technological, and patient concerns.

Legal and regulatory issues are waning because many states are addressing electronic business records, signatures, and record retention requirements. In fact, several recent federal regulations have explicitly supported more use of IT for health care.

Most state statutes are not very specific when it comes to EHRs, often citing in very general ways the need to address record authenticity, security, and confidentiality. States, as well as accrediting agencies, often rely on compliance with provider-developed policy to address retention and durability issues, storage safeguards, authentication requirements, protocols for assuring accuracy of entries, and data transmission integrity.

Check state statutes for:

☐ Record retention requirements

☐ Durability of record issues

☐ Storage safeguards

☐ Confidentiality provisions

☐ Authentication requirements

☐ Protocols for assuring accuracy of entries

☐ Data transmission integrity requirements

HIPAA Privacy and Security Rules go a long way to fill in gaps where state statutes are silent. Even though some states have more stringent requirements for some aspects of privacy, HIPAA requirements are generally broader in scope, while being very supportive of exchanging patient medical record information (PMRI) with others who have legitimate needs for the information.

States have recently been very active in updating their statutes, partially to align with HIPAA or assure even greater protection, while still facilitating entry into the electronic age. It is a good practice to work through your state medical society and/or legal counsel to be sure you have the most current picture. For example, the requirements for adopting standards for e-prescriptions under the Medicare Prescription Drug, Improvement and Modernization Act of 2003 (MMA) are leading to a number of states rethinking their requirements with respect to content and signatures for prescriptions.

Technology barriers should not be dismissed in evaluating EHRs. Although technology has come a long way, issues still remain with melding older and newer systems, interfacing systems from disparate vendors, finding the right HCIs, ensuring fail-safe measures, and myriad other considerations. Such technology issues are important to understand and address, but they should not deter a practice from moving forward. Many providers have opted to "wait for the technology to improve." The cycle of change in technology is as rapid as 18 months, and it often takes 18 months to select and implement an EHR, so there will always be newer technology available. Planning for obsolescence is considered essential by some; at a minimum, you should plan for continual improvement but not let the fact that there will be something newer on the market tomorrow deter you from achieving benefits today.

Patient response to adoption of EHR may be surprising to a practice. In general, most find that patients are very supportive; depending on your patient population, however, there may be specific and focused concerns. Certainly patients with especially sensitive conditions want to be assured you are protecting their privacy and the confidentiality of the information they supply to you. It may be necessary to step up your privacy measures even beyond those required by HIPAA to ensure that inappropriate actions don't speak louder than your words. Some providers, however, find that for some patients, interaction with the provider through the computer can enhance their willingness to share sensitive information. Appropriate expectations and boundaries must always be established.

Be aware that many stereotypes are not holding up. For example, many older patients do, in fact, use the Internet. Even if they are not themselves users, they are certainly aware that computers are important tools in everyday life. Similarly, the once frequently discussed "digital divide" between those who can afford computers and those who cannot is not as divisive as in the past; computer kiosks in public areas are becoming increasingly available and often provide recorded messages for poor readers as well as various language aids for those whose second language is English. Patients see computers used at their pharmacies and grocery stores, among other places, and recognize them as normal ways to do business.

Just as patients may come to expect your use of computers, they also expect seamless use of computers. They may be willing to accept a system being down occasionally or some other minor glitch, but be unwilling to tolerate intrusive downtimes. In fact, as you implement your EHR, you may want to tell your patients about its benefits and ask them for their patience. Be aware, though, that patients also can be very demanding when they understand what computers are truly capable of doing. Some of your patients may be more computer savvy than you are or ever want to be. Just as with any other new procedure, medical device, or therapeutic regimen you deploy, you must not be sloppy about your EHR implementation. This is no longer a back-office tool that probably doesn't matter to your image. Indeed, the EHR can be a powerful incentive or disincentive for patient satisfaction.

Resistance to Change

Resistance to change within the practice remains as probably the single greatest barrier in adopting EHRs, and requires the utmost attention. Identifying needed changes and seeing that they can actually be achieved through an EHR can best be accomplished through a number of measures:

▶ *Recognize the need for change.* Conduct an open dialogue with everyone in the practice about what the pain points are that are driving you to consider an EHR. Even for a large practice, it is important to ensure that everyone is aware of – and can contribute to – the business reasons for implementing an EHR. Once problems are recognized (and potentially documented because they can serve as a good start for developing a list of needed functionality for inclusion in a request for proposal [RFP]), it is important not to create a situation that assigns blame and fosters negativity. If a problem exists, address it and move on.

▶ *Fix problems unrelated to IT before implementing technology.* Remember the old computer adage, "garbage in leads to garbage out." An information system can help you to work smarter and more productively, but it cannot fix problems beyond those directly related to processing raw data into useful information. If the practice has staffing problems, personnel problems, attitude problems, customer service problems, or other such issues that you believe could negatively impact successful EHR adoption, fix those problems first.

▶ *Focus on a vision.* In the ideal scenario, the practice should create a vision of how IT might work and what it might accomplish. This is an ideal situation because very often members of the practice will have seen EHR systems demonstrated at professional meetings, read about them in the literature, or heard about them from colleagues. Such information can potentially bias a vision, so it is also important to bring knowledge and understanding of an EHR to the process of creating the vision, or it can become unrealistic. Again, active involvement of all members of the practice, working as a team, can help overcome any individual bias, create a strong vision and achieve a buy-in from all.

▶ *Commit to disciplined growth and development.* Once the vision is established, the practice must next find the most appropriate solution and work with it to achieve the anticipated benefits. This means that choices will have to be made. There are literally hundreds of EHR vendors, many potential migration paths and numerous approaches to an EHR. Although you don't have to investigate every possible scenario, you should consider a sufficiently broad spectrum of marketplace review and potential options. You may need to make compromises so the practice achieves the most for its investment. Once a commitment is made, the members of the practice team must do their part in making it work.

▶ *Celebrate success.* Implementing an EHR does mean change. It also means a degree of tedious work and some trial and error. Cultivate the virtues of maintaining an open mind, patience, and goodwill, and keep them constantly in the forefront as the EHR is implemented. Celebrating various milestones of success can go far in overcoming any of the irritations and setbacks along the way. This might include providing certificates for completion of training, a pizza party, thank you notes, or other tokens of appreciation.

▶ Planning for Selection and Implementation

To summarize, the steps to EHR selection and implementation involve:

1. Understanding the evolution of the EHR to appreciate the strategic options for and components that make up an EHR;
2. Recognizing benefits and ROI opportunities from an EHR;
3. Managing change required to achieve those benefits;
4. Determining your specific objectives;
5. Planning a migration path for the achievement of your specific objectives;
6. Determining your specific requirements for an EHR to convey to a vendor;
7. Organizing the selection and implementation effort;
8. Selecting the right vendor and application;
9. Planning and carrying out the implementation; and
10. Ensuring ongoing maintenance and enhancements for benefits realization and continual improvement.

► Conclusion

This chapter has addressed the key preparatory elements of understanding the EHR, including its variants, benefits, and barriers. EHRs are systems – with both animate and inanimate components. The animate components are probably the most critical and deserving of your attention, even though cost and activity will center around the inanimate components!

NOTES

1. Collen, MF. *A History of Medical Informatics in the United States, 1950 to 1990*, Indianapolis, IN: American Medical Informatics Association, 1995.

2. For example, the Integrated Health Association, a California collaborative initiative of Aetna, Blue Cross of California, Blue Shield of California, CIGNA HealthCare of California, HealthNet, and PacifiCare (www.iha.org).

3. HIPAA Privacy and Security Rules, 45 CFR Part 160, 162, and 164.

4. Amatayakul, M, SS Lazarus, T Walsh, and CP Hartley, *Handbook for HIPAA Security Implementation*, Chicago: AMA Press, 2004.

5. Waegemann, CP, "EHR vs. CPR vs. EMR," *Healthcare Informatics*, May 2003, pp 40-44.

6. Amatayakul, M, *Electronic Health Records: A Practical Guide for Professionals and Organizations*, Second Edition, Chicago: American Health Information Management Association, 2004 (www.ahima.org).

7. Health Level Seven, Electronic Health Record – System Functional Model Draft Standard for Trial Use (www.hl7.org).

8. Institute of Medicine, *The Computer-based Patient Record: An Essential Technology for Healthcare*, Washington, DC: National Academy Press, 1991, 1997. (www.nap.edu).

9. National Committee on Vital and Health Statistics, Letter to the Honorable Tommy G. Thompson on the Issues Related to the Adoption of Uniform Data Standards for the Electronic Exchange of Patient Medical Record Information, February 27, 2002 (www.ncvhs.hhs.gov).

10. Markle Foundation, *Connecting for Health: A Public-Private Collaborative*, The Personal Health Working Group Final Report, July 1, 2003 (www.connectingforhealth.org/resources/generalresources.html).

11. ASTM International, E31 – Continuity of Care Record (www.astm.org).

12. eHealth Initiative, "Electronic Prescribing: Toward Maximum Value and Rapid Adoption," Washington, D.C.: eHealth Initiative, April 14, 2004 (www.ehealthinitiative.org).

13. Berner, ES. *Clinical Decision Support Systems: Theory and Practice*, New York: Springer-Verlag, 1998.

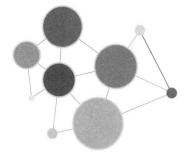

► TWO

EHR Technology

Chapter 1, Introduction and Rationale for EHRs, described the EHR as a system comprising hardware, software, people, policies, and processes. The people and associated policies and processes are indeed the most critical elements for an EHR to be successful, but the hardware and software – or technology – is what drives policy and process changes that result in successfully achieving the benefits for people.

EHR technology can be quite sophisticated – even the least sophisticated EHR products are not applications you buy at the local computer store and spend an evening loading and learning. EHR purchases require informed decision making. Implementation may require a vendor's or information technology (IT) consultant's assistance to help install, design screens and reports, and test the system, as well as to assist in training on the many nuances of its applications. Although those involved in making the selection decision or using the EHR do not have to be IT professionals, they do need an appreciation for the EHR technology to ask the right questions, get the right product, and understand how it can best work for your group. A basic understanding of EHR technology will also help in maintaining the system over time as well as help you anticipate when you may be ready for upgrades and enhancements.

THIS CHAPTER SERVES as an EHR technology primer. If you have a solid IT background, you may just want to skim the chapter to gain an appreciation for EHR configuration. If you have no IT background, however, the chapter is a "must-read" to learn the basics. Specifically, the chapter helps you:

▶ Understand the basic hardware components of EHRs;

▶ Evaluate various human-computer interface (HCI) devices for data capture;

▶ Explore networking and communication capabilities for sharing data internally and externally;

▶ Learn about the various operating system platforms on which EHRs are built;

▶ Recognize the various types of application software that make up an EHR;

▶ Appreciate the standards you should look for in an EHR to ensure interoperability with other systems;

▶ Understand how data are managed within a database and how to access that data;

▶ Appreciate the standards you should look for in an EHR to ensure data comparability; and

▶ Establish security measures to protect confidentiality, ensure data integrity, and support continual availability.

▶ Hardware

Hardware refers to the computer equipment on which the EHR runs. It includes computers to store programs and process data. Hardware also includes devices for entering and retrieving data (HCI devices); printing and incorporating paper documents into the EHR (printers, electronic faxes, scanners, document imaging systems); sharing data with other computers in the practice or from outside the practice (networking); and transmitting information to others (communications).

Computers to Store and Process Data

Today's EHR systems are generally built by using client/server architecture. This means that several computers are connected to one another, each with certain types of functions. Exhibit 2.1 provides an illustration of client/server architecture as well as other concepts of a network.

EXHIBIT 2.1 **Network Diagram** 1011010010100101001000010001100

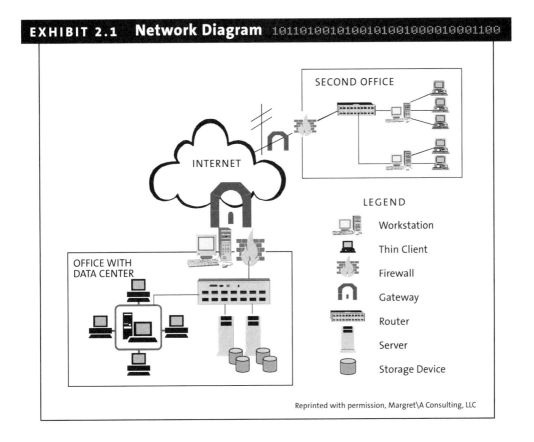

SECOND OFFICE

INTERNET

OFFICE WITH
DATA CENTER

LEGEND

Workstation

Thin Client

Firewall

Gateway

Router

Server

Storage Device

Reprinted with permission, Margret\A Consulting, LLC

Servers are computers that physically look no different from any other computer, but they contain more storage capacity and have faster processing capability. This means that the central processing unit (CPU) of the server computer needs to be as fast and robust as possible. The more random access memory (RAM), the more powerful and faster the server can be. Some servers include monitors to review system activity; others contain only the system unit. A small practice may have one server that maintains the application software and much of the EHR data. Larger practices may need more than one server, and still larger practices will often need several servers. When there is more than one server, the servers are networked to one another. Servers may be dedicated to specific functions, such as filing ("file server"), processing faxes or e-mail ("fax server" or "e-mail server"), or directing printers ("print server"). EHR vendors can provide advice on whether more than one server is necessary to optimize the use of their EHR products.

Because most EHR systems generate a significant volume of data, storing that data may be the function of yet another server or, for very large practices, even a separate storage network that provides special archiving, security, and disaster recovery capability. The storage network will include not only storage servers but also other types of storage devices.

If the practice has multiple locations, servers do not have to be present in every location. In fact, the more common approach is to have a central data center or IT department that maintains the server or servers for all locations. Each practice location is then connected to the central data center by using various communications capabilities.

Servers also do not necessarily have to be owned and/or operated by the practice. Some groups prefer to subscribe to an application service provider (ASP), a company that manages and distributes applications from a central operation. In this arrangement, the group pays a monthly fee to have its EHR software and data hosted by the ASP. Another alternative is for several groups of providers to jointly own and manage a central hosting center – spreading the cost across multiple entities. Chapter 6, How to Select the Right Vendor and EHR for Your Practice, discusses economic considerations for buying your own servers or using an ASP.

Other storage media that practices should consider are portable storage devices. These include floppy disks, CDs, DVDs, and USB drives, among others. All are useful, but also pose a greater security risk.

The elements known as clients include computers that are workstations, sometimes called "thick clients" or "fat clients," or computers that have been stripped of storage and processing capabilities, often called "thin clients." Chapter 7, Planning and Initiating an EHR Implementation, discusses thick and thin clients in detail.

In general, a workstation is a personal computer (PC) that may be a desktop or portable (e.g., a laptop, notebook, or tablet PC) model. A workstation provides input, output, processing, and some data storage. Data stored on a workstation may include certain files the user wants to be stored only on the workstation (for privacy or other reasons), or data stored temporarily by the computer itself during processing of the centrally stored application. For example, if you use the EHR and also manage quality assurance, you may want to store the quality assurance reports only on your own workstation. However, when you use the EHR, the computer will likely be temporarily storing some of the data as you capture and use it, and then sending it to a file server after you are finished. The section on Security in this chapter discusses the advantages and disadvantages of saving data to your own workstation.

PCs stripped of all but minimal processing and storage capability, or thin clients, depend on the servers in the network to perform their processing functions and store data. Thin clients are generally lower in cost than thick clients because they don't have all the functionality of the thick client. Thin clients are also generally considered more secure because they do not permit downloading of data onto portable storage media or transmission of data except through the central servers. This reduces the likelihood of stolen data, and it greatly reduces the potential for introducing viruses via portable storage media. However, not all EHR application software is designed to work well on thin clients. In addition, some thin client users find a small amount of lag time in processing data because there is no local processing capability. Groups should carefully weigh the pros and cons of thick vs. thin clients before deciding what to buy. It may also be possible to buy some of each. A key consideration, however, should be whether the EHR application software will run on thin clients.

Prior to the advent of client/server architecture, mainframe computers were used to store and process data, and "terminals" were connected to the mainframe computers as HCI devices. These terminals had no storage or processing capability. Thin clients are somewhat similar to these old terminals, but not quite because they have some very limited storage and processing capability to meet internal processing requirements.

Human-Computer Interfaces

HCIs are the devices used by people to enter and retrieve data. In the past, these were called input and output devices, or "user interfaces." The new term, human-computer interfaces, emphasizes the important role they play in gaining user adoption of the EHR at the point of care. Providers often specify preferences for HCIs, and they may not be the same for every person or setting.

Monitors and keyboards are the most common HCIs for retrieving and entering data. A provider may want a workstation for his or her office and the practice's reception area, but find a notebook or tablet computer more suitable for use in examining rooms. Monitors, keyboards, and notebook computers can be wall-mounted, secured to a cart, suspended from a ceiling, or built into a desk or table (recessed).

Mobile professionals introduce another situation to consider – portability. Many providers thought that personal digital assistants (PDAs) would be the answer to this problem, but they are finding the small screen constraining. In addition, software must be contoured to display on the PDA screens. PDAs with mobile phones offer the benefit of having only one device to manage, but many find it inconvenient to talk and review what is on the PDA at the same time, or they find they must always use a hands-free device. Older mobile phones may impose the risk of electromagnetic interference. If your practice uses electronic medical devices, such as infusion pumps or respirators, this may be a consideration. Tablet PCs are becoming very popular because they offer more "screen real estate" while being relatively mobile. The power source for all of these devices is another consideration. Most run on batteries, so battery life is a consideration. Connectivity is yet another issue. Some PDAs and tablet PCs dock into a workstation to download data for the day's patients; others have wireless cards that connect them to file servers as part of a wireless network. Although wireless devices introduce security issues (see section on Security in this chapter), those that do not store data have less of a security risk if the devices are removed from the practice and lost or stolen.

There are also choices of monitor style. Flat-panel monitors fit into tight spaces, but are generally more expensive than traditional ones. Large-scale monitors may be needed in certain situations, such as reviewing X-rays or some highly complicated sets of data (e.g., the status of every patient in an emergency department). A touch-screen monitor is also an option.

The type of keyboard must also be considered. Keyboards may be accompanied by a mouse, touchpad, or other navigational device – often there are personal preferences here as well.

In addition to the more traditional monitor/keyboard and navigational devices are special types of HCIs for certain circumstances. Many providers thought speech recognition would be a panacea for data entry. These devices have taken a long time to mature to the point that they capture a high percentage of what is said, but many providers now realize they are uncomfortable dictating into them in the examining room. Speech recognition devices, as well as their cousin, handwriting recognition devices, must be "trained" by users to recognize their particular speech or handwriting patterns. Any errors made by the system must be corrected – either by the user during the entry process, or later by a "correctionist." (Often transcriptionists who formerly transcribed dictation now make corrections in data entered through speech or handwriting recognition devices. Such a process, however, reduces the savings afforded by direct data entry by the clinician.) Most speech recognition systems simply result in an image of text – not discrete structured data that can be processed. However, there are also systems in which speech is used to select discrete data (instead of using a mouse or touch screen). Speech recognition systems also require faster, more powerful computers, and generally cannot be used with a thin client.

More sophisticated input devices might include digital cameras and video cameras, which may be suitable for certain types of specialists. For example, a dermatologist may want to take digital pictures of a patient's skin condition over the various phases of treatment. Or a physiatrist may want to use a digital movie camera to capture the gait of a patient before and after physical therapy. Digital pictures and digital movies can all be stored electronically.

The decision as to what HCIs to adopt must be made in concert with what the EHR application software supports, although most EHR software supports a wide range of such devices. The important point is that "one size does not fit all," even within one practice for one provider. It is entirely likely that different HCIs will be needed in offices, examining rooms, registration areas, conference rooms, and back-office departments. Use the checklist provided in Exhibit 2.2 on the next page to help you decide which HCI is right for each application and location in your practice.

Hardware for Managing Paper

Although you will want to reduce paper handling as much as possible when the EHR is implemented, there will always be some need for printing and for incorporating paper documents from other sources into the EHR.

► *Printers* obviously produce paper copies. Choices generally include laser or ink-jet, then black-and-white or color, and finally special features such as continuous-feed, label creation, and duplex printing. Laser printers produce the highest quality printed image and generally are more costly to purchase and operate than ink-jet printers. Black-and-white laser printers are less expensive than color laser printers. Unless you print some of your own brochures or patient instructions that may benefit from color enhancement, you probably do not need a color laser printer. The quality of ink-jet printers varies, with some rivaling the print quality of laser printers. They are generally less expensive than laser printers and offer color or black-and-white printing. Ink-jet printers are generally sufficient for most provider practices.

EXHIBIT 2.2 Human-Computer Interface Checklist 000010001100

HUMAN-COMPUTER INTERFACE	PRIMARY APPLICATION	LOCATION(S)
❏ Monitor		
❏ Traditional		
❏ Touch screen		
❏ Flat panel		
❏ Large scale		
❏ Keyboard		
❏ Navigational device		
❏ Mouse		
❏ Touch pad		
❏ Other:_____		
❏ Workstation		
❏ PC		
❏ Thin client		
❏ PDA		
❏ Notebook		
❏ Tablet		
❏ Mounting		
❏ Wall mounted		
❏ Ceiling mounted		
❏ Cart secured		
❏ Recessed		
❏ Speech recognition		
❏ Handwriting recognition		
❏ Digital camera		
❏ Digital movie camera		
❏ Other:_____		

Reprinted with permission, Margret\A Consulting, LLC

Some practices, however, may find value in acquiring a special feature printer. If your practice prints large batches of documents, such as claims, you might want to buy a continuous-feed printer. However, many practices are moving to electronic claims processing and no longer have need for such a printer. Special label printers are also available. If your practice does a lot of mailings, this may be useful. Bear in mind, though, that most standard laser and ink-jet printers can also be purchased with attachments that can provide these functions. Your volume should determine whether you need a dedicated printer to perform a specialty function. Another potentially useful feature is duplex printing, which prints on both sides of the paper. If you plan to continue to print everything from the EHR, storage costs can actually increase because the volume of material to be printed will increase. A duplex printer will cut that storage in half. Still, not printing the contents of the EHR on a routine basis will result in savings not only in printing and storage costs but also in costs associated with chart pulling and filing.

Printers are also available with fax and scanner functions. These printers can be useful if the volume of work associated with any one of the functions is low. If your practice receives many faxes or wants to scan all paper documents into an EHR, however, a separate fax machine and/or separate scanner will be necessary.

▶ *Fax capability* is also available electronically. Today you can purchase services that permit faxes to be directed to your e-mail account, accessible from your workstation. These can then be moved directly to an EHR (without having to scan a faxed document into the EHR). Faxes that do not relate to an EHR can be routed electronically to the appropriate person, printed, or deleted. Electronic faxes (e-faxes) eliminate paper clutter around a fax machine, and the ability to automate routing enhances productivity. The security of the fax is determined by the security of your e-mail server and Internet Service Provider (ISP).

▶ *Scanners and document imaging systems* also help you manage paper. The term "scanner" usually refers to a device that simply creates an electronic image of a paper document that you must then route to the appropriate place (e.g., an EHR, billing system or Microsoft Word® document file).

Document imaging is the term generally used to describe a comprehensive system in which paper forms are labeled with identifying bar codes for indexing purposes, and then scanned into a computer that captures the image of the form and uses the bar code for later retrieval. Depending on the extent of indexing, work queues can be created that notify various areas about work to be performed. For example, all new encounter forms can be queued for review by the billing staff. Yet, those encounter forms are still accessible should they need to be reviewed, such as if a pharmacy calls to check on a prescription. Automated creation of work queues is referred to as work flow functionality. For example, a notification can be placed in a provider's workstation in-basket regarding which documents require a signature. Once the document is signed, it can be routed to the EHR archive. Similarly, a document that must accompany a claim can be routed to the billing system for electronic or paper attachment.

Document imaging systems can also be integrated with other systems to receive output from them for incorporation with the scanned documents into an image repository. This is called a COLD (computer output to laser disk) feed. For example, if the practice has a laboratory information system or is electronically connected to an external laboratory that can send results electronically, it is possible for the lab results to be directly stored on the practice's laser disk storage system. It then becomes a part of the document repository and can be flagged in a provider's workstation in-basket for review.

Several products on the market today described as EHRs are essentially document imaging systems. These systems primarily afford easy access to content that was originally generated on paper. A document imaging system, though, still depends on the original use of paper to capture data, and hence it does not provide interactive decision-making support at the point of care. For example, a document imaging system cannot "read" the paper entry for a drug and offer a more therapeutically appropriate alternative or alert the prescriber that the patient is allergic to an ingredient in a drug being ordered. Because document imaging systems do not provide this level of clinical decision support or other complex processing capabilities, they are not technically considered to be EHRs. Exhibit 2.3 compares scanning, document imaging, and EHRs on key capabilities.

EXHIBIT 2.3 Scanning vs. Document Imaging vs. EHR 010001100

KEY CAPABILITIES	SCANNING	DOCUMENT IMAGING	EHR
Creation of content	Paper	Paper	Direct entry
Entry of data	Scanning	Imaging and COLD	
Timeliness of access	Delay during scanning	Delay during imaging	Immediate
Retrievability	Generally via one document at a time	Via content as indexed	Direct via any query
Accessibility	Viewable by multiple persons	Viewable by multiple persons	Viewable by multiple persons
Correction	Generally via printing and rescanning, or scanning an addendum	Potentially via electronic signature authentication	Direct via entry
Alerts and reminders	Only via notes made in documents	Potentially through work flow capability if data are entered and indexed	Direct through rules engine

Reprinted with permission, Margret\A Consulting, LLC

Networks and Communications

As illustrated in Exhibit 2.1, sharing data with other computers in the practice or outside the practice (networking) and transmitting information to others (communication) are critical technical components of any information system (IS).

Networking is achieved via a variety of network devices so that users can share data. As you purchase computers for your EHR, you will need a network interface card (NIC) or network adapter associated with each device to be included in the network. Each device must also have network operating system (NOS) software to manage the networking functions. Usually, at least one other device connects with all other devices and serves to route communications. A variety of these types of devices, such as routers, hubs, bridges, switches, and multiplexers are available. Which of these devices is used depends on the size and complexity of the network.

Finally, devices in a network must be connected for communications to occur. These communications connections may be restricted to only those between the devices in the practice, in which case the network is considered a local area network (LAN). Communications may need to occur within each of several locations of the practice and across the practice locations; this may require a wide area network (WAN) configuration. Many practices, whether using a LAN or WAN, also want connectivity with the Internet. Generally, three options are available with respect to how the connections are made to conduct the communications:

1. *Hardwire* (e.g., cabling or telephone wires) is generally the most expensive and difficult to install, but it is the most secure connection. Speed of transmission through cable or telephone lines depends on the type of service purchased.

   ▶ Cabling may be "dedicated" or "leased." When you install your own cable in a practice or between buildings, the cable is said to be dedicated. Unless the building in which a practice is located is already wired, pulling dedicated cable through walls and ceilings or floors is an expensive proposition. Laying cable from one building to another is an even more expensive proposition. Such cable, however, can produce very fast transmissions and, because it is dedicated, it is very secure. Leased cable services are now being offered by a number of companies. Such a service has become more popular since speed of transmission has been boosted. Various complementary services and devices provide varying levels of security.

   ▶ Telephone lines provide an alternative to cable. All telephone lines are leased, and the degree of privacy and speed depends on the service leased. Connections dialed using a telephone ("dial up") and modem (device that converts analog signals to digital signals and back again) are the cheapest, but also the slowest and least secure. "Private" line transmission service can be purchased, increasing cost, speed, and security. Integrated Services Digital Network (ISDN) lines are all-digital telephone services. Digital Subscriber Line (DSL) is a relatively new technology that uses existing telephone network wiring through a single data channel. High-density phone lines, such as digital T1 lines are also an option, although these are generally for large organizations. Very large organizations may lease an entire T1 line, including 24 communication channels. Smaller organizations, such as physician groups, may be able to manage with leasing only one or a few of the channels on a T1 line.

2. *Infrared transmission* is a form of wireless transmission by which data are beamed from one device to another. Many handheld devices and notebook computers have infrared transmission capability. This form of network transmission requires an infrared receiver that is hardwired to the server that is to receive the data. The biggest issue with infrared transmission is that a direct line of sight must be maintained between the device and the receiver. As a result, the distance between the device and the receiver must be fairly short.

3. *Wireless connections* via radio waves are becoming increasingly popular. Wireless technology creates wireless local area networks (WLANs) that provide the ability to broadcast data from mobile devices to other networked devices almost instantaneously. Each device must have a wireless access card that uses radio waves to communicate with one or more access point units located throughout the practice location or building. Multiple and overlapping access points can be added to cover large areas and assure full coverage. Most wireless networks are based on the IEEE 802.11 standard, which provides a fast connection speed. Bluetooth is another standard for wireless networks, but at a much lower power level than 802.11, making it suitable for PDAs and other small devices within relatively close proximity and in areas where many wireless devices are being used simultaneously.

Internet connectivity and use is often a function to consider when planning networks and communications. Internet use is becoming very important for communications among providers, with patients, and for staff to access various important resources. In addition to an Internet use policy (see Exhibit 2.4 on the next page) that describes how the Internet may and may not be used from your practice, security considerations are vital to safe Internet use (see the section on Security in this chapter.)

Access to the Internet also brings with it access to e-mail. Due to privacy concerns, especially with regard to the Health Insurance Portability and Accountability Act of 1996 (HIPAA), the use of e-mail to exchange protected health information (PHI) is generally not advised. Exhibit 2.5 on pages 37–38 identifies some options to consider for the exchange of e-mail containing PHI.

Web-based portals provide a single point of access to relevant information. The access can be controlled by using various access and authentication

EXHIBIT 2.4 Internet Use Policy Components 010010000010001100

Users using [*Name of Provider*]'s information technology systems to access the Internet are representing the organization. As a result, users are expected to conduct all business on the Internet in a professional manner.

A. Occasional, limited use of [*Name of Provider*]'s information technology systems to access the Internet for personal use is permitted subject to other provisions of this policy and subject to other personnel policies.

B. [*Name of Provider*]'s information technology systems may never be used to access the Internet for any of the following or other related purposes:
   1. To discuss confidential information about [*Name of Provider*]'s operations, personnel, patients, services, or systems;
   2. To express personal opinions on political, social, racial, religious, sexual, inflammatory, or other volatile subjects;
   3. To engage in exchanges of taunting, threatening, sarcastic, or otherwise hostile language with another Internet user;
   4. To download or display any pornographic or sexually explicit image or document;
   5. To download copyrighted material without permission from the author;
   6. To play games or engage in chat sessions of a non-business-related nature;
   7. To download software from the Internet without prior authorization from IT Services;
   8. To knowingly violate the laws and regulations of the United States or any other nation;
   9. To impersonate another or mislead another about the user's identity; and
   10. To distribute "spam" e-mail messages.

C. Employees using [*Name of Provider*]'s resources to access the Internet must never access Internet services such as e-mail, bulletin board messaging, or chat-mode conversations using their organization User IDs.

[*Name of Provider*]'s information technology systems are subject to audit and monitoring for the purpose of detecting inappropriate or unauthorized use of systems and networks or data. [*Name of Provider*] reserves the right to inspect and exercise control over any and all of our information technology systems with or without prior notice. All user access to and usage of the Internet is subject to monitoring and random audit.

Reprinted with permission, Margret\A Consulting, LLC

security measures, and the information can be supplied by using the eXtensible Markup Language (XML) standard to encode documents, data, and transactions. XML is a language that allows users to encode, or "tag," information for interchange, storage, or display. This language integrates structured and unstructured data from disparate sources, creating a single Web browser-based point of access. Users do not have to learn new

EXHIBIT 2.5   E-mail Policy   0100101101001010010100100001000011100

OPTION	DESCRIPTION
Prohibition	Use of e-mail to send any PHI to patients or other providers could be prohibited by policy. This is difficult to enforce, but manageable in a small practice, where everyone understands the consequences.
De-identified with other providers	Exchange of health information between providers that does not contain any patient identifying information is not restricted under HIPAA. However, few circumstances probably exist in which health information would be exchanged in a de-identified manner (because most such exchange would be for the purpose of a specific patient referral).
Limited with patients	Some providers are comfortable exchanging a limited amount of PHI via e-mail with certain patients with whom they have made an agreement to make the exchange. The agreement should authorize the provider to send PHI via e-mail to the patient and establish the ground rules for such exchange. Generally, these rules would include limitations on what PHI may be sent, to which address, the content of the subject line, expectations for response time, and other special considerations. Such e-mail communications should be retained in the patient's health record.
Encrypted exchange	Although HIPAA permits PHI to be disclosed via e-mail if the message is encrypted, few providers and patients have the capability to encrypt messages. Incompatibilities exist with different forms of encryption as well, so until there is a common standard, this degree of security is difficult to achieve.

continued next page

EXHIBIT 2.5   E-mail Policy *continued*   010010100101001000010001100

OPTION	DESCRIPTION
Receipt from patients	Although receipt of e-mail from patients containing PHI is not a wrongful disclosure under HIPAA, providers should be cautious about receiving e-mail. First, any response would probably entail PHI. Although such a disclosure to the patient is not wrongful, the e-mail could possibly be misrouted or become corrupted, which would constitute a wrongful disclosure. Second, many patients forget that e-mail communications they send from employer workstations are not private, so the patient is at risk for disclosing information to an employer by virtue of such company policy. Finally, receipt of e-mail from patients without established ground rules could set unrealistic expectations for responses, putting the provider at risk for medical liability.
Through portal	A secure, Web-based portal is a good solution to the electronic exchange of PHI among providers and with patients. In order for patients or other providers to access PHI, you would need to grant them access privileges. At that time, ground rules for use of the portal can be established; these rules can also be posted right on the portal. Portals typically use Secure Sockets Layer (SSL) security protection (similar to Web-based businesses that receive credit card information for purchases).

Reprinted with permission, Margret\A Consulting, LLC

technology or navigate multiple systems to access and act on the exact information needed.

▶ Software

So far, we have primarily discussed the devices, or hardware, that make up EHR systems and the fact that software of various types is needed to operate a network and create a virtual private network (VPN). Software is the set of instructions that make computer devices process data in the manner desired. Software may also be called a "program" or "code." Writing the program to perform certain processes is called programming or coding. Software comes in different computer languages, with certain languages more typically used to write specific types of programs.

Importance of Software

As you evaluate various EHR systems, you will want to consider the type of programming language(s) used. Languages change over time. For example, Cobol is a very old programming language. No one programs new systems in Cobol anymore, but there still may be some old mainframe systems that use such software. In many cases, software languages have various versions (e.g., Microsoft Windows® 2003 is a newer version of Windows® 2000). Newer versions of software, however, are often backward compatible, meaning that software written with a newer version should work on an older version, but this should always be confirmed.

It is important that you have some understanding of software types and versioning to avoid buying systems with old, obscure, or proprietary systems. There are several reasons for this. One reason is that you may acquire a system and then a few years later decide to acquire another system that is complementary to the one you have. Many practices start out with a practice management system (PMS) and then decide to add an EHR system. Software that is incompatible will mean that the two systems will not work together. Another reason for being aware of the type of software is that there may not be many people who know how to program in the older, obscure, or proprietary software. As a result, if you need some modifications made to the system or you need to upgrade it, you would be totally dependent upon the one company from which you acquired the original system. If that company is too busy to help you, or too expensive, or it goes out of business, it will be difficult to find other people to help you.

There are two main types of software: operating system software runs the technical components of the computers, and application software provides the IS functionality.

1. *Operating system software* runs the technical components of computers. For this reason, operating system software is sometimes referred to as the "platform" on which the system runs. Typically, there are server operating systems, client operating systems, and, as previously mentioned, network operating systems. The same or different software may be used for each type of operating system.

Operating system software may be generic or proprietary. A generic operating system is one based on a commonly used standard. For example, a version of Windows (e.g., Win 95/98, NT, 2000, or XP) is commonly used for client operating systems, and in many cases server and network operating systems as well. Other generic server operating systems include UNIX, Linux, Novell, Sun Solaris, MacOS, and IBM AIX. Each type of operating system has certain inherent features. For example, Windows provides a graphical user interface (GUI) that many people know from PCs used at home with Microsoft Office® (for word processing, spreadsheets, and other functions) or Microsoft Explorer® to access the Internet. UNIX was developed a number of years ago but is still used to run many large computer systems. Linux is a newer operating system, considered to be an "open source" operating system because source code for Linux is freely available to everyone. (Linux is not a derivative or version of UNIX.)

Some practice management and EHR system vendors use proprietary operating system software. This means that only applications developed by that vendor can run on the proprietary operating system. Systems with proprietary operating system software may be inexpensive, but, as previously noted, their incompatibility can make it difficult to expand systems by introducing applications that run on standard operating system software.

2. *Application software* processes data in specific ways to perform specific functions. Although users can write their own application programs, application software for physician practice computers is generally licensed from a vendor. Application software provides billing services, scheduling tools, documentation functionality, and other services. Just as with operating system software, application software may be written using a standard software language or a proprietary software language. Today, Visual Basic, Java, C++, and HTML are common languages used in writing software applications for EHR systems. Once again, older, less common or proprietary languages may mean lower initial cost, but over time they can be problematic.

Standards for Interoperability

Some application programs come "bundled" together as a set of integrated programs, such as a PMS that includes a scheduling function, billing system, and accounting program. Sometimes, however, application programs are licensed separately and must have another, special program written to be able to share data. Although this is most often true when systems are acquired from different vendors, it is possible that one vendor may have different types of application software that are not necessarily integrated. The programming that helps different applications share data is called an interface. For example, if you obtain PMS software from vendor A and EHR software from vendor B, to get the two to share data, such as patient demographics from the PMS to the EHR or charges from the EHR to the PMS, will require an interface for data exchange. The ease with which the interface can be created depends on whether each vendor has used standard protocols.

The most common standard protocol for health care software applications is Health Level Seven® (HL7®). HL7 is called a message format standard because it defines how the content of a message to be sent from one system to another system should be structured. If both vendors use an HL7 message format structure, it is much easier to write an interface that will more seamlessly get the products from the two different vendors to share data.

DICOM, which stands for Digital Imaging and Communications in Medicine, is a message format standard for the exchange of images, such as X-rays. Many EHR systems are beginning to incorporate the ability to store and view digital images directly from within the EHR system.

Another important health care standard is that from the National Council for Prescription Drug Programs (NCPDP). This is a message format standard for use between retail pharmacies and payers. However, now that physicians are starting to use e-prescribing capability, the e-prescribing system must be able to transmit the content of a prescription from the device to a retail pharmacy using the NCPDPSCRIPT protocol. Because many medical group and hospital applications use HL7, the HL7 and NCPDP standards organizations are getting together to "harmonize" their standards so they use common structures and can work together.

Database Management Systems

Because EHR systems are used to manage large volumes of textual data, a special type of application software is generally used to help manage the data in a database structure. The software that runs these special databases is typically database management system (DBMS) software. Microsoft® SQL Server, Oracle, Sybase, Access, Cache, and DB2 are common examples of DBMS software. The databases for an EHR are usually set up so that there is a significant amount of preprogrammed data entry and retrieval functionality. Much of this can be tailored to meet the needs of various specialists. However, there are times when someone may want to make a special type of query into the database that is not preplanned by the vendor. Some DBMS software is more user friendly than others; in other words, some facilitate the retrieval of special queries on the database, whereas others require some programming knowledge to make the query.

Depending on the level of sophistication sought for your EHR, the database may be structured as a clinical data repository (CDR) used to organize data from multiple source systems (including a PMS and any other stand-alone systems, such as a laboratory information system, radiology information system, and so on) into a single database. (If there is no central repository, data from multiple systems must be interfaced, which could make the system complex to manage and/or unstable.)

As one uses the EHR, data are entered and retrieved from the CDR. Such entry and retrieval functioning is called online transaction processing (OLTP). This supports normal, day-to-day patient care services such as recording a history and physical exam, reviewing diagnostic studies results, updating a problem list, developing a treatment plan, and so forth. However, if you want to run a query to analyze a large amount of data in the repository, the analysis function can take a long time and can reduce the speed with which the system can respond to normal OLTP. If you intend to perform a significant amount of analysis on your data during normal hours, you may want to obtain a system that extracts data from the clinical data repository and puts it into a clinical data warehouse (CDW). The CDW can then be tapped for analytical processing, called online analytical processing (OLAP). For example, to develop your own clinical practice guidelines, you would run some highly complex queries to evaluate what treatment regimens would be most effective for a certain type of condition.

Data Comparability

A CDR serves primarily to pool data into one location so that different applications do not have to be used to retrieve enterprise data. However, the implications of such a repository go far beyond simply pooling data. Data that go into a repository need to be standardized; otherwise, the computer cannot make comparisons. A simple example would be data in metric form coming from one source and data in non-metric form coming from another source. Consider the impact this would have on the ability of the computer to evaluate a child's height and weight on a standard growth chart.

The purpose of ensuring that data are standardized is referred to as data comparability, which means that each data element has one meaning, known to all users. Data comparability may be achieved by using a common data dictionary. A data dictionary identifies the meaning of each data element to be entered into the EHR. Hence, the system would specify, for example, that height and weight need to be recorded in inches/feet and pounds/ounces. The data dictionary would also include a list of all the other terms used in the EHR and their meanings.

Exhibit 2.6 provides an illustration of a structured data entry screen. In this example, the physician is entering the history of present illness (HPI) for a patient, John Sample, who is being seen in follow-up to an old myocardial infarction (MI). The provider can simply check the various symptoms the patient may be presenting associated with chest pain, such as severity, change, activities, and so forth. Each of the descriptions would be listed in the system's data dictionary. In this particular system, as each data element is checked, a sentence is formulated by the system. For example, checking "mild severity" produces a statement that "Symptoms are described as mild." In this way, the provider can produce a summary of the patient's HPI in narrative form even though only a few keystrokes are required to check off the variables that describe this particular patient.

EXHIBIT 2.6 Structured Data 01011010010100101001000010001100

⌘ File Edit View SOAP In-Basket Tools Help	🕐 📄 ⏳ ☎ 📖
John Sample	CC: *Old MI*

🗂 CC	📂 HPI	🗂 PMH	🗂 FH	🗂 SH	🗂 ROS

Severity of Symptoms	Change in Severity	Patient cannot . . .
☒ Mild	☒ Stable	❒ Walk short distances
❒ Moderate	❒ Improving	❒ Walk long distances
❒ Severe	❒ Worsening	❒ Climb stairs
❒ Excruciating	◯ [ ]	⊙ [Swim more than 4 laps]

Symptoms are described as mild. Symptoms have been stable. Patient cannot swim more than 4 laps.

Reprinted with permission, Margret\A Consulting, LLC

In addition to checking the data elements that describe the patient's condition, most EHRs permit the provider to also enter unstructured data. This is important because potentially not every conceivable type of data to be recorded can be anticipated. However, it is difficult for unstructured data to be later processed.

In the example in Exhibit 2.6, if the physician wants to indicate that John Sample cannot swim more than 4 laps, this information can be entered into the box providing for unstructured data as cannot "Swim more than 4 laps." The computer will capture this data and place it into the narrative being constructed. However, if other patients also have difficulty swimming, but the physician records the findings as cannot "Sustain swimming for more than 10 minutes" or cannot "Do laps," the physician would not easily be able to find patients with old MI who had difficulty swimming because the data are not structured in the same manner. Even doing a word search on "swim" would miss the patient who was described as cannot "Do laps."

Clinical Decision Support

Although it may not have been the initial intent to use an EHR for analysis of data such as described above, one of the most valuable functions of an EHR is to provide clinical decision support (CDS). CDS is a function wherein patient-related information and clinical knowledge are intelligently filtered and presented at appropriate times to enhance patient care, provide patient safety, improve productivity, and assure appropriate reimbursement. The filtering process can be achieved by a rules engine, which uses special analytical processing tools to make comparisons and perform other logical processes on data. Most EHR systems come with a set of CDS tools that can be tailored to the needs of the clinicians.

For example, the rules engine could evaluate what is entered as the patient's chief complaint or reason for the visit and provide logical branching through questions that the physician has previously decided should be included in the history for such a patient. This set of questions is referred to as a structured data template. A rules engine would present the appropriate set of questions for a physical exam for a male vs. a female. A rules engine can be used to establish the minimum data that must be recorded for every patient, or every type of patient. For example, if the three elements shown in Exhibit 2.6 are deemed by the physicians to be required for every patient whose previous MI is being evaluated, the computer system could restrict the physician from moving to the next screen if something is not checked in each of the three boxes. Caution should be applied, however, in having too many such rules. Rules can distract the user from a thought process associated with a patient condition. Restrictive rules can be irritating to work with if they have to be frequently overcome for exceptions. Most clinicians find that judicious use of rules can be a very helpful aid.

Many EHR systems provide alerts when a drug is prescribed to which the patient is allergic, or when there is a contraindication between the drug being prescribed and a drug the patient is currently taking. Such a system can link to the patient's health plan and provide information about whether the drug is covered by the patient's specific benefits. In these e-prescribing examples, the EHR combines data previously recorded in the patient's record, such as allergies and medication history, with information from a drug knowledge base and a health plan formulary.

Another example of decision support is an Evaluation and Management (E&M) coding advisory function, such as illustrated in Exhibit 2.7.

EXHIBIT 2.7   Example of Clinical Decision Support   0000100001100

⌘ File Edit View SOAP In-Basket Tools Help   🕐 🗂 ⌛ ☎ 📖

John Sample	CC: *Old MI*

☐ E&M Advisor

Is visit primarily counseling/coordination?   ❏ Yes   ❏ No

What is type of patient?   ❏ New   ❏ Established   ❏ Consultation

What was amount/complexity of data reviewed?
  ❏ Review/order clinical labs
  ❏ Review/order radiology tests
  ❏ Review/order other dx or tx interventions
  ❏ Discuss test results with other provider
  ❏ Review old records or hx from another provider
  ❏ Review and summarize old records for another provider
  ❏ Independently review dx data

What is risk of complications?   ❏ Minimal ❏ Low ❏ Moderate ❏ High

This note is in compliance with CPT-99212
  Code: ❏ 99211   ❏ 99212   ❏ 99213   ❏ 99214   ❏ 99215

Reprinted with permission, Margret\A Consulting, LLC

All of the analytical and CDS functions illustrated depend on the fact that the data have defined meanings. Whereas some vendors supply a data dictionary for this purpose, as previously mentioned, many are beginning to implement standard vocabularies. What this means is that every data element presented in the structured data templates actually is represented by a standard vocabulary code that can be easily processed by the computer.

A standard vocabulary means that all data elements are defined not only within the one system, but across all other providers' systems. In this way, when a drug is ordered, it can, in fact, be compared to a drug knowledge base or health plan formulary. Standard vocabularies help providers share data with one another as well as across systems within one provider setting.

One of the most widely known and used standard vocabularies is the Systematized Nomenclature of Medicine (SNOMED®). Originally developed by the College of American Pathologists (CAP) as a clinical language standard, SNOMED has now incorporated a number of other, more specialized vocabularies to become internationally recognized as the most comprehensive reference terminology for all of medicine. SNOMED includes medical terminology, specialty terminology, nursing terminology, and many other important structures. The National Library of Medicine (NLM), which is a part of the U.S. Department of Health and Human Services (HHS), has licensed SNOMED for free distribution to vendors and providers. The NLM has also mapped SNOMED to Current Procedural Terminology® (CPT®) International Classification of Diseases (e.g., ICD-9-CM, ICD-10), and other classification systems. As a result, if all data entered into the EHR were represented in SNOMED, by using a decision support rules engine, the data could be filtered to produce CPT and ICD-9-CM codes automatically for billing purposes.

Obviously then, the more data that can be structured for data entry purposes, the easier it will be for the computer to process the data in various ways. However, depending on the nature of the patient's illness, type of documentation being performed, and the number and types of CDS rules, structured data entry can mean that documentation will take more time to perform (although it will be more complete). As a result, various forms of structured data entry have been developed to reduce data entry time. Exhibits 2.6 and 2.7 illustrate the use of pick lists that facilitate data entry. Another approach is through the use of "macros," sometimes called "smart text." Macros permit a user to enter a word, phrase, or even entire paragraph by just keying a few letters into the system. For example, a pediatrician can have a macro called "ear" for the common symptoms of ear infection. Typing "e-a-r" can produce an entire paragraph. There may then be just a few variables to enter, such as whether the ear infection is in the left or right ear and its severity. Some vendors have had success with combining speech recognition and structured templates by which, instead of clicking on each item, the selection can be spoken.

Other Tools

Finally, there are special types of tools, or toolsets, that can help to perform certain functions. These toolsets may be written in a special type of language or one that is the same as the DBMS. Some of these tools are developer tools, in the event you want to develop your own software or customize the software you have acquired. Caution should be applied, however, in customizing software yourself. First, some vendors will not give you access to the "source code" or the actual program that runs your applications. If you don't have this access, you will not be able to do any customization yourself. If you do have access to the source code, however, any customization you perform could nullify a maintenance contract with the company. You need to decide whether you want to take this risk because not having a maintenance contract may mean you won't get certain support you need when there is a problem. Even if access to the source code does not have an impact on the maintenance contract, it is possible that any upgrade the vendor supplies may not run properly because you have made changes that are incompatible with the upgrade. In this case, you will need to hire the vendor or someone else to "fit" the new software upgrade to your old, customized version. Still, it is a good idea to at least obtain the rights to the given source code in the event that the vendor goes out of business. This assures that you have the ability to maintain it through a third party, at least until you transition to a new system.

▶ Security

An important aspect of all EHR technology is security.[1] All security decisions should be based on a risk analysis that helps to determine the most appropriate controls for your environment.[2] An EHR certainly heightens security risk and the need for more advanced controls. The standards required under the HIPAA Security Rule provide a good starting point to check off what is needed. Exhibit 2.8 lists the HIPAA security standards.

EXHIBIT 2.8   HIPAA Security Standards   1010010100100001000110

SECURITY STANDARDS	CFR SECTIONS	SECURITY IMPLEMENTATION SPECIFICATIONS (R) = Required, (A) = Addressable
ADMINISTRATIVE SAFEGUARDS		
Security Management Functions	§164.308(a)(1)	Risk Analysis (R) Risk Management (R) Sanction Policy (R) Information System Activity Review (R)
Assigned Security Responsibility	§164.308(a)(2)	(R)
Workforce Security	§164.308(a)(3)	Authorization and/or Supervision (A) Workforce Clearance Procedure (A) Termination Procedures (A)
Information Access Management	§164.308(a)(4)	Isolating Health Care Clearinghouse Function (R) Access Authorization (A) Access Establishment and Modification (A)
Security Awareness and Training	§164.308(a)(5)	Security Reminders (A) Protection from Malicious Software (A) Log-in Monitoring (A) Password Management (A)
Security Incident Procedures	§164.308(a)(6)	Response and Reporting (R)
Contingency Plan	§164.308(a)(7)	Data Backup Plan (R) Disaster Recovery Plan (R) Emergency Mode Operation Plan (R) Testing and Revision Procedure (A) Applications and Data Criticality Analysis (A)
Evaluation	§164.308(a)(8)	(R)
Business Associate Contracts and Other Arrangement	§164.308(b)(1)	(R)

continued next page

Technical Security

With respect to EHR hardware and software, access controls are needed so that each user can uniquely identify himself/herself to the system and be provided with the appropriate privileges. Access control is usually accomplished through a unique user ID. The access controls should coincide with the minimum necessary use policies the practice has established under the

EXHIBIT 2.8   HIPAA Security Standards *continued*   0010000100001100

SECURITY STANDARDS	CFR SECTIONS	SECURITY IMPLEMENTATION SPECIFICATIONS (R) = Required, (A) = Addressable
PHYSICAL SAFEGUARDS		
Facility Access Controls	§164.310(a)(1)	Contingency Operations (A) Facility Security Plan (A) Access Control and Validation Procedures (A) Maintenance Records (A)
Workstation Use	§164.310(b)	(R)
Workstation Security	§164.310(c)	(R)
Device and Media Controls	§164.310(d)(1)	Disposal (R) Media Reuse (R) Accountability (A) Data Backup and Storage (A)
TECHNICAL SAFEGUARDS		
Access Control	§164.312(a)	Unique User Identification (R) Emergency Access Procedure (R) Automatic Logoff (A) Encryption and Decryption (A)
Audit Controls	§164.312(b)	(R)
Integrity	§164.312(c)(1)	Mechanism to Authenticate ePHI (A)
Person or Entity Authentication	§164.312(d)	(R)
Transmission Security	§164.312(e)(1)	Integrity Controls (A) Encryption (A)

HIPAA Privacy Rule. The minimum necessary use standard requires that categories of PHI and any conditions applicable to access be established for every class of user.

If your implementation of the EHR does not result in fully integrated applications, access controls will need to be applied for each application. Unfortunately, this can require logging in and out of applications as they are used. This situation should obviously be avoided if possible, but if not possible, the unique user ID and password (for authentication) should be synchronized so they are the same, or single sign-on technology should be considered. Single sign-on technology provides a single point of entry to otherwise disparate applications.

Because access controls limit access to those with a treatment, payment or operations reason for access, the HIPAA Security Rule also requires that there are emergency access procedures in place if another provider must take over a patient's care or some other extenuating circumstance requires access that is not normally permitted. Such emergency access procedures are often called "break-the-glass," and operate with much the same philosophy as associated with fire alarms. Emergency access procedures should be very easy to invoke (such as through entry of a special password or by identifying the reason for the access from a drop-down menu). Emergency access should also generate an audit trail that is reviewed by a supervisory person or the patient's primary physician. Emergency access procedures are as much a strong deterrent as they are a facilitator to gain necessary access.

Audit controls provide for a record of access. They should be used not only for recording emergency access, but for documentary evidence of access and accountability. Audit controls are required by HIPAA. Some vendors provide highly detailed audit controls, indicating what data were accessed and what function was performed (e.g., view only, entry of data, correction of data, print, and so forth.). Each group should determine the extent of audit controls reasonably needed in the practice based on the risk that there may be inappropriate access from inside the practice or hackers attempting access.

Data integrity controls protect data from inappropriate alteration or destruction. Data integrity controls are highly technical, performing checks on the data as they are processed or transmitted. Most EHR vendors can advise you on the controls they have in place and can suggest whether you need to complement them.

Authentication is the verification that a person or entity (such as another computer system) seeking access to data is the one claimed. Whereas the access control identifies the user in relation to privileges (through a unique user ID), authentication proves the user is really the user. The simplest form of authentication is a password. Users must use their own passwords to access a system or the authentication process will not be accomplished. Because passwords must be memorized, people often create simple passwords associated with things they will remember such as birthdates or pets' names. As a result, these passwords can be easily guessed. Passwords that are more difficult to remember are often written down, and ultimately these can be found. Because weak passwords or password practices create vulnerability, many EHR vendors are encouraging the use of a token, often in combination with a password, or biometrics to ensure that one's authentication is not being spoofed. Even if you believe your practice staff are above using someone else's password, they are one of the easiest means for a hacker to gain access to your systems. Providers should also recognize that as EHRs are used to record all clinical data, including prescriptions, it is essential to have the accountability afforded by unique user identification and authentication.

Transmission security, sometimes called network security, refers to protections when data are transmitted from within your entity to another entity or when you receive data from another entity. For example, if you electronically exchange data with a hospital, commercial lab, other providers, and health plans, you will want to evaluate how the transmission is secured. This may be via dedicated cabling or telephone lines. When using the Internet, a virtual private network (VPN) may be necessary. This is essentially the creation of a private tunnel through the Internet via software. A VPN can be thought of as a special envelope that protects the content of a message as it moves through the Internet. VPN software can be loaded to your own network, or you can subscribe to a VPN service. One or more firewalls may also be needed. A firewall is a device that examines traffic entering and leaving a network and keeps some types of traffic from passing from one network, such as the Internet, to another network, such as your LAN, based upon a set of rules.

As wireless networks gain in popularity, it is important to recognize that they have their own special security risks as well as large returns on investment (ROIs). Wireless devices permit mobile health care professionals to take devices with them from examining room to examining room, from practice site to hospital and from bed to bed, and even to connect remotely. However, wireless sniffers can fairly easily listen to transmissions; spoof addresses; steal identities; and reroute, jam, or flood traffic. When considering a wireless network, it is important to understand the latest technology and make informed choices. Today, Wi-Fi Protected Access (WPA) is a new wireless security standard based on the IEEE 802.11i wireless security protocol. This standard provides authentication, temporal key integrity, and message integrity checks, all of which are based on strong encryption methodologies. The world of wireless is an extremely dynamic one, with improvements being made constantly. As you consider deploying a wireless network, conduct a comprehensive site survey to determine the intended coverage area, research the latest types of equipment, use directional antenna and careful channel selection, and always reset the manufacturer's default settings to your own.[3]

Electronic Signature

In general there are three forms of electronic signatures that may be used by a medical practice:

▶ Digitized signature;

▶ Electronic signature; and

▶ Digital signature.

A digitized signature is an image of an original pen-to-paper signature, or wet signature. A digitized signature is considered the least secure and is usually not used in an EHR setting.

On the other hand, an electronic signature is generally used form of authentication that only the computer user knows, such as a password and/or token. This is the most common form of electronic signature and is generally accepted in most states for all legal documents except prescriptions for controlled substances.

Finally, a digital signature is a form of encryption that not only provides authentication (identifying "who" the signing person is) but also non-repudiation (proving the person is the one who is claimed). Because digital signatures are not yet required by law and are not interoperable among systems, they are not widely used except within a large network or clinic group.

Physical Security

In addition to the technical security measures just described, physical security measures are very important. These include facility security, device and media control, and workstation use and security.

Most practices already address many physical facility security measures. Certainly doors are locked and smoke detectors installed. Most building codes require a minimum of security measures before you can even operate a medical practice. Many of these security measures, however, are intended to address personal safety. It would be prudent to review physical facility security from the perspective of information security, especially when implementing an EHR. Servers and other devices associated with more robust networks and more workstations often need greater protection. Instead of storing these in the back of an office, it may be necessary to devote a separate, locked room for them. Many providers use closets for this purpose – although there needs to be sufficient air circulation to prevent power problems. Other power considerations are also important, so consider surge protectors, uninterruptible power supply (UPS) systems, and back-up generators.

As devices become smaller and more portable, they also become much more prone to loss or theft. Each practice should have an inventory of all devices containing PHI, and staff should be trained to be alert to their absence. It may be necessary to bolt devices to furniture. Consideration should be given to removing the capability to store data on the hard drive and/or memory of any devices, including workstations and portable devices. Data stored to the hard drive of a workstation may not be backed up when the network storage server is backed up, so data can be lost forever if the workstation crashes or is stolen. Sometimes it is tempting to store especially sensitive information only on a workstation. This temptation, however, should be translated into stronger access controls so the data can be adequately protected and backed up. Many wireless devices can be used solely as input and output devices, with any data that are temporarily kept in the device's memory for processing purposes being wiped out when the device is moved out of range of a wireless access point.

When data are stored on portable storage media, the media also should be protected. If you back up onto tape or laser disks, these should ideally be stored in a separate, and protected, location. There should be policies for not permitting anyone to bring media into the practice, at least not without clearance from someone who has checked it for problems. For example, loading a pretty screen saver from a CD could introduce a virus. It could also be the means for someone to copy and remove data from your practice. Therefore, even if the medium has been approved for use, it should be installed by the practice manager or IS staff and then be removed from the premises immediately. This is one of the reasons thin clients have become popular – they do not have floppy or CD drives. However, if your EHR requires a true workstation, the external drives can still be disabled.

Workstation use and security have been alluded to when Internet use and e-mail were described. Such use policies, however, should not be restricted solely to the use of the Internet. Exhibit 2.9 on the next page provides examples of policy statements that are appropriate for the internal use and security of workstations.

EXHIBIT 2.9   Workstation Use and Security Policies 00010001100

The following uses of workstations are explicitly prohibited:

A. Use that impedes, interferes with, impairs, or otherwise causes harm to the activities of others, such as by "resource hogging" or "spamming." Knowing or reckless distribution of unwanted mail or other unwanted messages. Other behavior that may cause excessive network traffic or computing load.

B. Use that is inconsistent with [*Name of Provider*]'s non-profit status, such as use for commercial purposes, endorsement of any political candidate, or ballot initiative.

C. Harassing or threatening use, such as by the display of offensive, sexual material in the workplace, or repeated unwelcome contacts with another person.

D. Use damaging the integrity of [*Name of Provider*] or other information technology systems. This includes the following:
    1. Attempts to defeat system security (e.g., by "cracking" or guessing and applying the identification or password of another user or compromising room locks or alarms);
    2. Unauthorized access or use, including deliberate and unauthorized changes to data or applications, "promiscuous" network monitoring, or tapping data or voice lines;
    3. Disguised use, such as masquerading or impersonating others;
    4. Distributing or launching computer viruses or other forms of malware;
    5. Modification or removal of data or equipment without specific authorization; or
    6. Use of unauthorized devices, such as attachment of any external disk drive, printer, video system to [*Name of Provider*]'s information technology systems.

E. Use in violation of civil or criminal law – such as promoting a pyramid scheme; distributing illegal obscenity; receiving, transmitting, or possessing child pornography; infringing copyrights; and making bomb threats. Users should be aware that copyright law governs the copying, display, and use of software and other works in digital form (text, sound, images, and other multimedia).

F. Use in violation of [*Name of Provider*]'s contractual obligations, including limitations defined in software and other licensing agreements and those associated with external data networks when using such networks.

G. Use in violation of any other [*Name of Provider*] policy, including, but not limited to, those regarding sexual, racial, and ethnic harassment as well as work-unit policies regarding incidental personal use.

Reprinted with permission, Margret\A Consulting, LLC

Remember that workstations, other devices, electronic media, and paper are also candidates for redeployment or disposal at some point in time, and therefore should be reused or disposed of in a secure manner.

Administrative Security

Just as with physical security, most providers have some administrative security policies already in place. For example, you may already be monitoring IS activity to prevent virus and other malicious software attacks, or you may be monitoring Internet access to ensure that you are provided the speed and bandwidth you are paying for.

Some special security concerns exist with respect to EHRs. This is especially true in the area of contingency planning. Even if you continue to print out the content of the EHR and file paper copies, it is very likely that the EHR is your primary source of information and you would be hard pressed or highly inconvenienced if the system were down for any period of time. Once you become paperless, which surely ought to be one of the goals of an EHR system, it is absolutely critical that you have not only backup copies of your system and data, but also backup devices that permit you to continue processing with backup data. Unfortunately, because the cost of an EHR is relatively high, many providers seek to trim costs where they can. Fully redundant system capability and backup should *not* be one of these areas. The components of a contingency plan for an EHR should include:

▶ *Backup Plan.* This plan should specify how backup is performed, what is backed up, the media on which backups are stored, where backups are kept, and who has access to the backups. For a paperless environment, backup should be performed simultaneously with use of the system, not simply each evening or once a week. The backup should be performed not only to a set of backup media (redundant array of inexpensive, or independent, disk, or RAID, is often used to create EHR system backups) but on a second complete system. This is often called a fully redundant, or mirrored, backup system. Consideration should be given to having a third backup performed to media that can be removed and housed elsewhere, or transmitted to a remote location. This is especially true for practices that are located in any area where there are significant weather and other types of threats that can destroy computer systems. You should have a backup not only of the data but the system itself. This is especially true if you have tailored your system with special data entry templates, CDS, and so forth, which most practices do. Backups can be stored on stationary or removable hard drives, tape drives, or CD-ROMs, or, as noted above, transmitted to a remote backup service. A distinct chain of command for who has access to the backups should be in place, and all in the chain should practice performing the backups and recovering with the backups.

▶ **Disaster Recovery Plan.** This plan extends your contingency plans beyond just the backups. You possibly have a disaster recovery plan for your practice already. If not, the EHR should trigger creating one that covers all components of how and when to declare a disaster, who will do what in a disaster, and how to recover from a disaster – including relocating to temporary quarters, protecting your practice and the data during the recovery process, contacting insurance companies and working with local authorities.

▶ **Emergency Mode Operation Plan.** This plan refers to how you will continue to operate in the event of an emergency that wipes out part of your computing capability, but is not of a disaster scope that would put you out of business. Some practices are investigating reciprocal agreements or business continuity plans by which computers can be run from a remote location. This might be a second location owned by the practice; the local hospital; or even a local school, bank, or other business.

▶ **Testing and Revision Procedures.** These procedures are critical to ensure that your plans work as expected. All too often, the first time a plan is tested is when it is needed, and unfortunately the test fails. It is a good idea to conduct "disaster drills" with your backup, disaster recovery, and emergency mode operation plans. Procedures and technology used in the contingency plans must be reliable and easy to use.

In addition to these components, contingency plans should ensure flexibility as use of the system grows.

It is very important that the security measures described here be included in your questions to ask vendors because they are requirements under HIPAA's Security Rule. Some vendors may be in the process of adding these functions, and you should determine when they will be made available as part of the regulatory upgrades to the system.

▶ Conclusion

This review of EHR technology should serve as a guide as you evaluate all aspects of acquiring an EHR. Many providers look at the functionality but not beyond to the technical platform being used. Although functionality is critical to day-to-day utilization of the system, the technical underpinnings can mean the difference between a solid investment and a poor one.

NOTES

1. Amatayakul, M, SS Lazarus, T Walsh, and CP Hartley, *Handbook for HIPAA Security Implementation*, Chicago: AMA Press, 2004.
2. Amatayakul, M, and SS Lazarus, *Complete Guide to HIPAA Security Risk Analysis: A Step-by-Step Approach*, New York: Brownstone Publishers, Inc., 2004.
3. Retterer, J, and BW Casto, "Practice Brief: Securing Wireless Technology for Healthcare," *Journal of AHIMA*, May 2004 – 75/5.

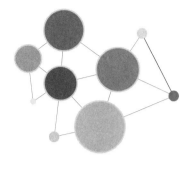

► THREE

Determining Your Group's Objectives

The previous chapters discussed the wealth of terms and types of systems that may be considered an EHR and the full scope of technology that may be associated with an EHR. Now you can consider how your practice plans to implement an EHR, what components you actually need and want, and over what timeline you want to achieve your ultimate goals and objectives.

The approaches to implementing an EHR are varied. Some groups may be inclined toward a "let's try the least sophisticated" approach first. Other groups may feel they are ready to "go for the most comprehensive." Still other groups may want to pick and choose among various applications. Many groups start out thinking they want to "go paperless" or "go digital," but may not have thought about the full range of possibilities. Advanced planning can help in making informed and judicious choices. In general, it is best to decide upon a migration path that reflects current readiness and capabilities, short-term objectives, and longer-term goals. Just as there is no one EHR system, there is no one "right" answer to achieving the EHR for everyone (no "one size fits all").

THIS CHAPTER HELPS you to determine your group's readiness, overall goals, and objectives, and hence the scope of an appropriate EHR. Specifically, the chapter helps you:

► Understand the level of benefits that may be achieved based on the level of EHR sophistication acquired;

> ▶ Determine the group's readiness for various components of an EHR;

> ▶ Reach consensus on EHR goals and objectives;

> ▶ Identify considerations that should be made based on the size and specialty of the group;

> ▶ Organize the EHR planning effort; and

> ▶ Plot a migration path from your current position to where you plan to be in the future.

▶ EHR Benefits Matrix

As shown in the previous chapters, a group can't just go out and buy an EHR – the acquisition of an EHR is not the same as buying software from the local computer store and implementing it out of the box. Adopting EHR functionality involves many steps and much planning.

Among the first steps should be understanding the level of sophistication for which your group is ready. Exhibit 3.1 illustrates the types of applications, corresponding technology, and respective benefits in increasing levels of sophistication. Recognize, however, that this is the "30,000-foot picture" of the EHR. The intent here is to gain an overarching understanding of the general type of system the practice is interested in acquiring. Chapter 5, Determining and Managing Your Requirements, identifies specific and detailed functionality.

Pathway for Groups New to Computers

In considering the type of information system (IS) for a practice that is new to computer usage, you may want to start at the first level, where access to data is enhanced. This may mean you acquire clinical messaging capability, a provider portal, or at most a document imaging system. Even this first step requires careful planning because once providers perceive the benefits of data availability and their own enhanced productivity, they often want to move forward rapidly to other aspects of the EHR. For such a group, a basic data access system should lead smoothly to the more sophisticated levels of technology. For example, if your timeline is anticipated to be short, clinical messaging may be a good start that enables migrating to the work flow and documentation steps. However, if your timeline is anticipated to be longer because clinicians are less interested in a point-of-care application, a document imaging system may afford the data availability

EXHIBIT 3.1 EHR Benefits Matrix 1010010100101001000010001100

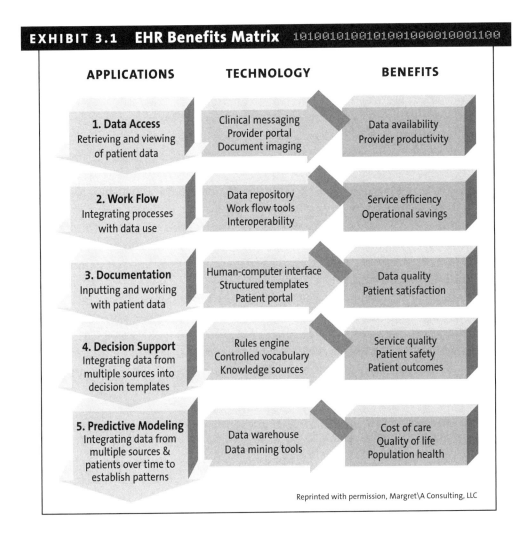

Reprinted with permission, Margret\A Consulting, LLC

and work flow that are appreciated for many years to come. Clinical messaging systems are generally less expensive than document imaging systems, which require a fair amount of investment. The clinical messaging system can also be continued simultaneously with other levels of sophistication, whereas document imaging (for all but a few documents requiring a wet signature, which can just as easily be accomplished with a scanner) would generally be replaced when moving to a system that includes point-of-care documentation through structured templates.

Pathway for Groups with Computer Expertise

If your group already has a practice management system (PMS) or other clinical information system support, and providers are accustomed to using computers at home or even spreadsheets or databases in the practice for tracking certain information, you may be more ready for an EHR that encompasses several, if not all, of the levels of applications and their technology. The mere capability to access data can impact work flow. If document imaging is chosen, you will see that many work flow support tools are associated with it. However, many practices may feel that document imaging only perpetuates the paper environment. In this case, documentation will contribute significantly more to changes in work flow and processes.

For example, in the past when a handwritten prescription was handed to a patient, in 30 percent of the cases the practice could anticipate a telephone call from the pharmacy for clarification.[1] With e-prescribing, fewer communications will result from legibility problems. If e-prescribing is coupled with eligibility and benefits information obtained through the e-prescribing tool, fewer calls about potential changes due to a patient's health plan requirements will result. Access to drug knowledge coupled with medication history from both the health plan and the practice's own EHR can contribute significantly to identifying contraindications. Finally, if the dispensing pharmacy is able to send information to the provider about the fill status of the prescription, the provider can follow up on potential compliance problems.

Another example of work flow and process changes with a huge impact are those associated with billing and collections. The Health Insurance Portability and Accountability Act of 1996 (HIPAA) standards for electronic transactions and code sets were intended to provide administrative cost savings. Unfortunately, only the standardized electronic claim has been rolled out in most provider settings – at a cost, rather than at a benefit. But adding an EHR to the practice can support a significantly greater amount of administrative and financial support. With an EHR in place, practices will be able to turn to an eligibility inquiry for all patients to ensure co-pays and deductibles can be collected; to claim status and remittance advice transactions to reduce billing costs; and ultimately, to electronic claims attachments to reduce copying expense and delays. Payers are starting to recognize the importance of supporting these transactions in a more robust manner.[2] Coupling these transactions with enhanced Evaluation and Management (E&M) coding support through the EHR should yield significant benefits in cash flow, time savings, collection fees, and revenue optimization. These benefits are achieved, however, only if steps are taken to ensure that the work flows and processes to support them are in place.

▶ EHR Readiness

The readiness assessment in Exhibit 3.2a may help organize your thinking about which EHR scenario is best for your group. This assessment is designed to ensure that each question is read and answered independently of the others (hence, the most positive response is not always "strongly agree").

EXHIBIT 3.2a   EHR Readiness Assessment   0010100100001000110

☐ PHYSICIAN ☐ NURSE ☐ OPERATIONAL STAFF Concerning EHRs . . .	STRONGLY AGREE	AGREE	NEUTRAL	DISAGREE	STRONGLY DISAGREE
1. They increase practice efficiency.					
2. They are not as secure as paper records.					
3. Our patients are expecting us to use them.					
4. They will improve my personal productivity.					
5. They are difficult to learn how to use.					
6. Their use in the examining room is depersonalizing.					
7. Their cost is beyond our budget.					
8. They improve quality of care.					
9. They reduce staffing requirements.					
10. Computerized alerts can be annoying.					
11. We are in an age where we must exchange data electronically with other providers and payers.					
12. Medicine is too complex anymore without access to evidence-based support.					

Reprinted with permission, Margret\A Consulting, LLC

The responses to the EHR readiness assessment are intended to be mapped to the levels of sophistication in Exhibit 3.1. Tally the number of responses in each cell. Once you have made this tally, look at where most of the results fall. Consider the following list, which relates to the 12 assessments in Exhibit 3.2a, in interpreting your group's readiness for an EHR:

1. There should be fairly strong agreement that practice efficiency is improved before ever considering an EHR. Because some work flow improvements can be effected before provider documentation, agreement with this statement is important for both data access and work flow levels of sophistication.

2. EHRs can be made more secure than paper records. Because the level of security is often a misperception – and sometimes even an "excuse" for not implementing EHRs – any disagreement with this statement needs to be addressed before an EHR is acquired.

3. EHRs can be used "behind the scenes" for both access and documentation, but patients are likely to become increasingly aware of them when they are used for work flow and definitely at the documentation level of sophistication. A positive sense of patient interest is important, although some patients assume that providers make greater use of computers today than are actually made, so in some respects responses to this question are more reflective of the need to overcome provider resistance than patient resistance.

4. Agreement regarding personal productivity is important. Some providers have "heard" that using a computer takes longer, especially for documentation. Although some documentation may take slightly longer than handwriting or dictation, the downstream time savings are immense. For example, EHRs save providers' time in not having to sign dictation after the fact or having to respond to telephone calls because information was not recorded or is illegible.

5. Some skepticism about the difficulty of learning to use an EHR is healthy; and being overconfident of one's ability to learn to use an EHR can actually work against its adoption. Any set of middle-of-the-road answers to this question is generally considered a good sign of readiness.

6. This question about depersonalization is similar to question 3 about patient expectations, except it generally is more focused on the doc-

umentation aspect of EHRs. Strong agreement with this statement should alert you that providers are not confident in their computer skills. However, strong agreement can also suggest that it is important to find the most appropriate human-computer interface (HCI) and work processes that do not necessarily force a provider to use the computer in the examining room. Depersonalization can be overcome by engaging the patients in their use (such as showing patients graphs of their vital signs or changes in their lab results).

7. A healthy skepticism about cost is also important. It may be necessary to look at responses to this question in light of other responses. Sometimes cost can be used as an excuse not to acquire an EHR for other reasons. However, if all other indicators are positive, the cost factor is probably an accurate reflection of true financial concerns. Alternatively, an unrealistic cost picture can simply mean a lack of education. Costs of EHR systems can vary widely. The least sophisticated systems cost the least, but this can be somewhat deceiving because the return on investment (ROI) then is generally also low. Sometimes a somewhat more costly system actually has a much greater financial benefit. Furthermore, depending on how quickly the practice wants to move through the levels of sophistication, a lower-cost EHR may end up costing more in retrofitting additional applications.

8. Improvement in quality of care is probably the primary long-term benefit of an EHR. However, quality-of-care benefits exist by merely having the chart always accessible. Quality-of-care benefits are enhanced as one moves along the migration path, so the stronger the agreement with this question, the more likely the practice is interested in pushing through the levels of sophistication.

9. Healthy skepticism about staffing is also important. In general, vendors will attempt to sell EHRs on the basis of staff reduction. In reality, existing staff are redeployed to other tasks. In smaller practices especially, the only staff reduction might be in reduced overtime or usage of temporary staff. Larger practices may see some potential for staff reduction in clerical support and transcription services. Actual reduction vs. redeployment is an important factor to discuss, and something to which planning should be directed.

10. Provision of alerts is an inherent (but not the only) part of clinical decision support; but some skepticism is also appropriate here. It

has been found that too many alerts can be disruptive and even hold some potential for liability if too much reliance is placed on them. However, judicious use of alerts, especially those that operate in the background and provide for optional use, are powerful aids. Negative responses here would suggest that the migration path be extended to allow sufficient time for earlier phases to create interest in and desire for more clinical decision support.

11.   Cautious optimism might be the best response about exchanging data electronically. Obviously, electronic claims and other such transactions are part of HIPAA, and many providers are engaging in those transactions already, potentially with some improvement in work flow.[3] Planning is necessary to ensure that more comprehensive data are exchanged when there is a legitimate need among authorized parties, or when data are truly de-identified for use in predictive modeling.

12.   Cautious optimism is probably also the best response to the last question on evidence-based medicine. Responses may vary by specialty. Certainly, agreement is a strong indicator that the value of an EHR is understood, especially supporting the more sophisticated phases.

To help you understand your group's perceptions, use the map shown in Exhibit 3.2b. For example, if most responses to the first question clustered in the Strongly Agree and Agree areas, then your group is ready for data access) and work flow (applications 1 and 2 in Exhibit 3.1), as also stated in item 1 in the list above. For large groups, you might consider separately tallying responses from each type of potential user (e.g., physicians, nurses, operational staff).

▶ Consensus on Goals and Objectives

A readiness assessment tool such as provided in Exhibit 3.2 can be a useful way to gain consensus on goals and objectives and highlight where pockets of resistance may still need to be overcome. The tool is especially useful because it avoids "group think" or any sense of coercion from a member of the group who is especially in favor or opposed to an EHR.

When bringing the results to a meeting of the group, take care not to reveal the identity of any individual's responses. The purpose of the assessment is to educate and inform the group as a whole on what level of sophistication

EXHIBIT 3.2b   **EHR Readiness Assessment Map**   0010000100001100

(Numbers in cells correspond to the level of sophistication in Exhibit 3.1)

☐ PHYSICIAN ☐ NURSE ☐ OPERATIONAL STAFF Concerning EHRs . . .	STRONGLY AGREE	AGREE	NEUTRAL	DISAGREE	STRONGLY DISAGREE
1. They increase practice efficiency.	1, 2				
2. They are not as secure as paper records.				1	
3. Our patients are expecting us to use them.	2, 3				
4. They will improve my personal productivity.	2, 3, 4				
5. They are difficult to learn how to use.			2, 3, 4, 5		
6. Their use in the examining room is depersonalizing.				3	
7. Their cost is beyond our budget.			2, 3, 4, 5		
8. They improve quality of care.	1, 2, 3, 4				
9. They reduce staffing requirements.			1, 2, 3		
10. Computerized alerts can be annoying.			3, 4		
11. We are in an age where we must exchange data electronically with other providers and payers.		3, 5			
12. Medicine is too complex anymore without access to evidence-based support.			4, 5		

Reprinted with permission, Margret\A Consulting, LLC

may work best. Much has been made of the importance of leadership involvement as a critical success factor in achieving the benefits of an EHR. If the leadership of the group is not behind an EHR, there may not be sufficient financial support to make it truly operational. There may also be greater willingness to run parallel systems to "accommodate" those who don't want to use a computer. Because such parallel systems are costly to maintain, the EHR will not be as successful as possible in achieving the anticipated ROI. Alternatively, however, a group's leadership should not force more on the overall group than they are ready to undertake. Extremely enthusiastic leaders may have to temper their goals to ensure buy-in from all. True leaders will use the results of this assessment not only to plan the appropriate level of sophistication but also to take special interest in addressing areas of concern.

Goals

Goals are the overall end result one hopes to accomplish by doing something. Goals should be established in advance of approaching EHR vendors, so that the group is not swayed by sales pitches. At a minimum, goals should address:

> ▶ *The ultimate level of sophistication desired.* A good way to describe this is by using the statements in the EHR Benefits Matrix in Exhibit 3.1.
>
> For example, the group plans to acquire an EHR in two phases. The first phase will provide enhanced data access (Level 1), and the second phase will integrate processes with data use to improve clinical work flow (Level 2) and provide clinical documentation support (Level 3).
>
> ▶ *The financial commitment.* This includes the amount and sources of funding willing to be made over the period of time in which the ultimate level of sophistication of EHR is achieved.
>
> For example, the group expects each partner to contribute $X in the first year to acquire basic hardware and software functionality for the first phase. Within M years, Y percent of the group's profits will be used to invest in the second phase of EHR implementation. Individual partners will be expected to invest on their own in any additional devices they wish to use for remote connectivity.
>
> ▶ *The desired benefits portfolio.* This especially includes specific quantifiable benefits, some of which should be financial and others of which may be qualitative.
>
> For example, it is expected that an N-year payback period will be achieved for the initial investment, and an M percent internal rate of return will be achieved on the second investment within Q years of implementing the second phase.

Objectives

Objectives are the key milestones the group expects to accomplish throughout its quest to achieve its goals. For example, objectives may:

► *Delineate a migration path* toward achieving the ultimate level of sophistication, identifying the specific sequence of applications and technology.

For example, the network will be upgraded to support N existing workstations, M workstations will be purchased, and a clinical messaging system will be acquired. E-prescribing tools will be acquired with a drug knowledge source and used independently to support improved patient safety. Work flow tools will then be used to integrate with the current PMS, and EHR software will be acquired to support structured templates for point-of-care documentation. Finally, a provider/patient portal will be created for secure remote connectivity, and electronic data interchange will be added to the e-prescribing capability.

► *Identify a timeline* for implementing each component and the expected benefits that must be achieved before progressing to the next stage of the migration path.

For example, the initial upgrade of hardware and software will start in year one. A payback period of N years is to be achieved primarily through improved managed care contracting due to demonstrable reduction of repeat tests as a result of availability of test results for every patient visit, as well as improved referral capability through being able to send chart information electronically to referred providers. The M percent internal rate of return in Q years will be achieved primarily through improved coding as a result of documentation prompts, elimination of transcription through direct clinician documentation, and further enhancements of managed care contracting through in-network referrals. In addition, patient satisfaction scores will increase to the S percentile through fewer billing hassles and improved prescription refill processing. Finally, no additional clerical staff will be necessary to support one additional nurse practitioner who will be added to support T percent growth in the number of patients that market demographics predict will be added to the caseload within Q years.

► *Establish expectations* for adoption of the EHR by all members of the group. This would include special considerations based on the size and nature of the practice.

For example, all family medicine providers should be using clinical messaging within X months of adoption, and all cardiology providers should be using clinical messaging within Y months of adoption. Within N months of implementing the second phase of the

EHR, paper chart pulls will be discontinued for all providers except for patients who have not been seen since the implementation of the EHR. Clerical staff will be deployed to abstract data from old charts into the EHR, and within the following M months all chart pulls will be discontinued. Providers who require further historical information on their patients will be required to pay for retrieval of the charts from a warehouse.

▶ Special Considerations

Note that in the examples provided, somewhat different expectations were established for different specialty groups. Depending on the size and nature of the group's practice, special considerations may need to be made in selecting and implementing an EHR. As a general rule the larger and more complex the practice, the more complex the EHR system. Exhibit 3.3 illustrates this relationship.

Size

The size of the practice obviously makes a difference in the complexity of the system, although not necessarily in its comprehensiveness. A practice of one, two, or three providers is less likely to have its own lab or other ancillary services, and therefore will not have to interface an EHR with such source systems. In this case, there generally is one practice within which to manage a network, very likely one hospital with which the providers are affiliated, maybe one external lab, and few other providers with whom to exchange data. Small practices generally do not become involved in clinical trials, training programs or other such potential uses of data from EHRs. A small group may not need the infrastructure of a full-time project manager or a formal steering committee to organize the EHR effort. Decision making is more centralized and less complex.

However, small provider groups potentially have the ability to adopt EHR systems that are quite comprehensive. Because the group doesn't have to bring along those who aren't as interested in an EHR as others, fewer compromises have to be made. Also, because the technical infrastructure is more contained and straightforward, resources can be focused on comprehensive functionality, if desired. Alternatively, processes in the practice may also be straightforward, not requiring the comprehensive support of a fully robust EHR. Whatever level of sophistication is chosen for the small practice, the importance of involving all stakeholders should not be dimin-

EXHIBIT 3.3   Determinants of EHR Complexity   0010000100001100

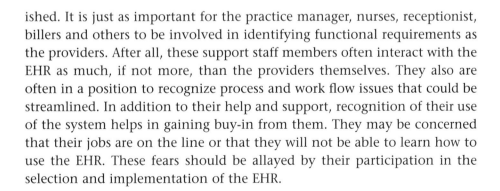

Reprinted with permission, Margret\A Consulting, LLC

ished. It is just as important for the practice manager, nurses, receptionist, billers and others to be involved in identifying functional requirements as the providers. After all, these support staff members often interact with the EHR as much, if not more, than the providers themselves. They also are often in a position to recognize process and work flow issues that could be streamlined. In addition to their help and support, recognition of their use of the system helps in gaining buy-in from them. They may be concerned that their jobs are on the line or that they will not be able to learn how to use the EHR. These fears should be allayed by their participation in the selection and implementation of the EHR.

A larger practice generally increases the complexity of the systems to be connected to the EHR. There potentially are more source systems, more than one site to be connected, and many more external providers with whom to connect than in a small practice. As more providers and other types of staff are involved, the complexity and formality of the decision-making process is increased, the need for formal project organization rises, and the need for consensus building becomes extremely important. In this case, every potential user may not be directly involved in the selection and implementation process, and continual awareness building and orientation are critical to achieving success.

Sometimes as a result of the complexity, the larger practice may decide to phase in an EHR or establish less sophisticated overall goals for itself. Benefits can be just as impressive, however, because larger practices tend to have a greater need for process improvement and work flow enhancements. Not every large practice, however, should consider the need to reduce its level of sophistication or lengthen its timeline for adoption. Much will depend on the current existence of computer use. In fact, many large practices may already have IS departments and highly sophisticated needs.

Specialty

The specialty of the practice can also impact EHR selection and implementation. In general, primary care providers find the work flow and decision support functionality of EHRs especially helpful. There is often more variability in the conditions they treat that may benefit from alerts and reminders, knowledge sources and coding support. Alternatively, single specialty practices may not need as much decision support, although this often depends on the actual specialty. Specialists who treat chronically ill patients may have needs very similar to those of primary care providers. Surgical specialists may have less need for decision support, but a greater need for connectivity to exchange data with referring providers and health plans, and more capacity to view and process images. Understanding your use of data currently and how you want to enhance that use should help you understand the level of EHR sophistication you may want to achieve.

Multi-specialty groups also have certain challenges. Just as there are generalists and specialists of many types in health care, there are also vendors in the marketplace that tend to either generalize or specialize. For example, some EHR products may originally have been developed by or for a cardiology practice, orthopedic practice, endocrinology practice, or obstetric practice – to name just a few of the more common types of specialty products. These products are ideal for those types of single specialty practices. They work less well for multi-specialty groups, although products of a more general nature may not have the level of sophistication desired by some of the highly specialized providers. Today, more vendors are recognizing the importance of providing customizability and specialty support, but some market differentiation still exists, and groups should consider this in their selection process. Identifying the original creator of the software the vendor is supplying can be a strong clue as to its specialty nature.

Community Served

The community served may be an important element for consideration. If the community is stable wherein patients are long term and providers get to know them better, less decision support may be required. But in communities where patients are more transient or where there are large companies that change insurance carriers and health plans regularly, there may be a greater need to exchange data with other providers, more unusual health problems and more need for reminders. A group practice affiliated with a medical school or a teaching hospital may be more inclined to do research and need the ability to manage clinical trials data. There may be special needs for countersignatures of trainees or educational support. A group practice in its own building may have different needs than a group practice in a large complex of provider practices where there may be some economies of scale available for network infrastructure or support. Recent changes to the Stark law against physician self-referral may facilitate community-wide information systems support.[4]

▶ Organizing the EHR Effort

The size and specialty of the group also determine the level of organization necessary to achieve the EHR. Small groups should not assume that no special organizational efforts are needed. Because the EHR effort is not small, even the smallest practice may find that they don't have time to adequately carry out the planning, selection and implementation details that make for a successful effort. Even though small practices do not need the degree of structure and formality a larger practice might, the suggestions in this section can be scaled so that all groups will benefit from some degree of organization.

Organizing the EHR effort often includes the following considerations:

> ▶ *Project manager identification.* A project manager is a person specifically appointed to be responsible for seeing that all the details of the EHR effort are carried out. This is an essential function that someone in the practice should assume (see also *Consultants and other resources,* discussed below). This does not

necessarily mean the project manager must install the hardware and software, but it does mean that there is an assigned individual responsible for monitoring all aspects of the EHR effort. Chapter 1, Introduction and Rationale for EHRs, provided a "job description" for a project manager who can successfully effect change. In a small practice, the role of project manager may have to be taken on by an existing staff member. If so, the practice should attempt to determine the number of hours per week this individual will need to spend and then make other staffing adjustments as necessary. The practice might have to introduce some part-time help. Such staff additions need to be factored into the overall costs associated with EHR implementation.

▶ *EHR planning team creation.* An EHR planning team is a group of individuals who represent all stakeholders in the practice. At a minimum, there should be a physician, nurse, operations staff member, and – if on staff – health information management (HIM) professionals (medical records), and IS staff members. In a very small group, every provider and staff member may be on the EHR planning team. A large group, obviously, will need to have representatives of each stakeholder type. The purpose of the planning team is to ensure that all aspects of the EHR are considered in planning, selecting, implementing, training, and ongoing use. In larger groups, it is wise to include some curmudgeons or other skeptics – for whom participation will be as much a way to represent their interests as to educate and hopefully convert them. The planning team is often chaired by the project manager, although it could be chaired by a member of the group's management team, using the project manager more as an internal consultant. In very large groups, there may be a steering committee whose role is to provide oversight and approval, as well as an EHR planning team that performs more of the specific functions described above.

▶ *Consultants and other resources.* Consultants and other resources are often used for a variety of purposes in planning and implementing an EHR. Whatever the size of the group, it may be beneficial to engage a consultant for specific tasks if no member of the group has that special expertise, if there simply are not enough staff resources, and/or if an unbiased, neutral third party is needed to facilitate decision making. Consultants can be very helpful in assessing a group's readiness for an EHR, clarifying goals and objectives, conducting operations and work flow analysis, identifying a suitable set of vendors to consider, managing vendor selection and contract negotiation, and aiding in implementing the system. A consultant can be also used as a project manager. In whatever manner a consultant is used, it is important to be very specific about the consultant's duties, responsibilities, and authority. In addition, a consultant must transfer applicable knowledge to the group's staff so they can become self-sufficient. Because vendor selection may be a one-time event, it is not necessary for staff to become expert in this process. Various parts of system building and training activities, however, are tasks of an ongoing nature, and staff members should learn to do this on their own.

Other resources that may be utilized include legal counsel to review contract terms and compliance issues, a financial auditor or advisor to assess availability of capital and recommend sources of funding, and security experts to assess system vulnerability to attack. In considering other resources, the group should also identify the availability of internal resources, what additional resources may be needed, and how to acquire them. In some cases, a group may find it necessary to add an IS analyst and/or network technician. Other options include using an application service provider (ASP), remote connectivity option (RCO), or outsourced services. Chapter 6, How to Select the Right Vendor and EHR for Your Practice, further describes these options.

▶ Migration Path

Once an EHR project is under way, documenting a migration path and establishing standards requirements are important functions. A migration path can help you:

- ▶ Clearly see a logical flow of sophistication and requirements for each level;

- ▶ Identify costs and benefits of each phase and overall;

- ▶ Explain the goals and objectives of the EHR to everyone in the group;

- ▶ Serve as a springboard for determining the requirements that you present to vendors; and

- ▶ Stay the course, especially when tempted to make costly deviations over time.

A migration path is simply a plan that describes how you will get from where you are today to your ultimate goal. Exhibit 3.4 is a useful way to document your migration path. You may construct the migration path in any form you might find useful, but using a matrix structure helps to plot various factors to consider across a timeline. Important factors to consider include what applications will be needed; what is the nature of the database, knowledge sources and standards to be applied; what networking and other technical infrastructure elements are needed to support the applications and database structure; what HCIs will be deployed; and what operational issues must be addressed. The first part of the migration path should reflect your current state. Then you can identify the objectives and components for each phase. Some groups may want to simply number the phases; others may want to specify dates associated with each phase.

The level of detail you record in the migration path is up to you. It generally is determined by the extent to which you want to control your EHR environment. Some groups may want only to identify applications and operational issues, leaving the more technical aspects of the plan to a consultant and/or vendor. Other groups may want to describe generically the technical aspects of the plan and leave specifics to a consultant and/or vendor. The more you know about information technology (IT), the more inclined you may be to add specificity. However, being too specific can also lock you into a configuration that might not allow you to take advantage of certain vendor offerings. Flexibility is probably the best approach in constructing this plan: Identify what you think you want, get help from a consultant or vendor, modify the plan, and continuously document your current state so you have a basis for subsequent planning.

Applications Description

The first step to constructing your migration path is to list all applications currently in use. If you have a PMS, it is a good idea to list the major functions it performs because not all PMSs include the same functionality. Then, when identifying the applications to implement over future phases, you will recognize what applications you have to build upon, what you may need to replace, and what may be missing and must be included in subsequent phases. For example, your group may have started out with a billing system, and then added a PMS for appointment scheduling and encounter management. Depending on the EHR components you acquire next, you may want to upgrade the billing system or replace it with one that is integrated within the EHR. Identifying applications across a planning horizon will help ensure that they are implemented in a logical manner.

EXHIBIT 3.4   EHR Migration Path 11010010100101001000010001100

(Examples shown in italics)

	TODAY	PHASE 1	PHASE 2	PHASE 3
Objectives		1. Data Access	2. Work Flow 3. Documentation	4. Decision Support

Applications	▸ *Billing system*
	▸ *PMS:*
	  • *Appointment schedule*
	  • *Encounter management*
	▸ *Dictation system*
		▸ *Clinical messaging*
		▸ *E-prescribing (formulary access)*
			▸ *Provider portal*
			▸ *Structured templates*
			▸ *Work flow tools*
			▸ *E-prescribing (connectivity)*
				▸ *Rules engine*
				▸ *Patient portal*
				▸ *E-prescribing (CDSS)*

Database, Knowledge Sources and Standards	▸ *HL7: PMS billing system*	▸ *Drug knowledge base*	▸ *Report writer* ▸ *DMBS* ▸ *ASTM CCR* ▸ *Rx-Norm* ▸ *NCPDP SCRIPT*	▸ *Clinical data repository* ▸ *AHRQ clinical guidelines* ▸ *CMS medical quality indicators*
Network and Other Technical Infrastructure	▸ *LAN* ▸ *Modem (1)*	▸ *Intranet* ▸ *Firewall* ▸ *Access control* ▸ *Authentication*	▸ *WLAN* ▸ *Scanner* ▸ *RAID backup* ▸ *Database server*	▸ *PACS* ▸ *Network attached storage*
User Interface	▸ *Desk top PCs* ▸ *Black and white dot matrix/ inkjet printers*	▸ *Workstations* ▸ *PDAs* ▸ *Color laser printer*	▸ *Tablet PCs* ▸ *Speech recognition*	▸ *High-resolution monitors*
Operations	▸ *Practice manager* ▸ *Maintenance agreement* ▸ *Contract transcription* ▸ *Contract billing*	▸ *IS technician* ▸ *EHR planning committee* ▸ *Physician Champion* ▸ *Internet Service Provider*	▸ *Web consultant* ▸ *EDI consultant* ▸ *Phase out transcription* ▸ *Phase out paper-based records* ▸ *Reciprocal backup site*	▸ *Paperless practice*

Reprinted with permission, Margret\A Consulting, LLC

Database Structure, Knowledge Sources and Standards Description

Database structure refers to how your data are managed within the system. You may want to identify at what point you will consider the database as the primary source for clinical data and the legal medical record. If there is special functionality to be acquired relative to the database, note this here. For example, acquisition of report writer software to create customizable reports, a clinical data repository (CDR), a clinical data warehouse (CDW), and data mining tools would be listed here. You may or may not want to specify the type of database management system (DBMS). As noted in Chapter 2, EHR Technology, the most common databases for EHRs include versions of either Oracle or Microsoft® SQL. However, as you review potential vendors, you may want to determine their DBMS in relationship to your capabilities and overall goals. For example, if a vendor indicates it uses DB2 for its DBMS, you may want to look for a vendor that uses more current tools. You might have staff members who know Microsoft Access®, but this may not be sufficient if your long-term goal is to ultimately have a clinical data repository. If the vendor uses a little-known DBMS, it may be more difficult to get help over time, especially if the vendor goes out of business.

Knowledge sources are resources that help you use the more sophisticated EHR functions. They are typically acquired through subscription services or other external resources.

A rudimentary e-prescribing system provides access to one or more formularies that may be supplied as part of your payer contracts. You may currently have some of these on paper, or you might have access to some via a Web site. Such formularies, however, will eventually be available for downloading to the EHR or e-prescribing device.

Drug knowledge base subscriptions supply information beyond just a list of drugs approved by a payer. Cerner Multum, First Data Bank, and Medi-Span are among the most common vendors of drug knowledge bases.

Clinical practice guidelines and quality indicators help enhance structured templates and build a clinical decision support (CDS) system. EHRs usually contain a starter set of templates, and you may prefer to modify these or build your own. There are several sources of clinical practice guidelines. The Agency for Healthcare Research and Quality (AHRQ) and the Centers for Medicare and Medicaid Services (CMS) Medical Quality Indicators are widely used knowledge sources. The Physicians' Information and Education Resource (PIER) from the American College of Physicians provides evidence-based clinical guidance available as a freestanding resource on the Web and on personal digital assistants (PDAs). PIER is designed to integrate with EHRs.

Standards are prescribed ways of doing things that ensure universality. Standards typically used in EHRs include message format, or "interoperability," standards, and vocabulary, or "comparability," standards. Chapter

2, EHR Technology, provides technical information about standards. It is a good idea to specify that the EHR should be compliant with certain standards because such compliance makes them easier to use, enhance and add to over time.

▶ *Interoperability standards* are protocols that define how data are structured and formatted to ensure that the data can be exchanged between information systems – whether within the practice or externally with other practices. For example, Health Level Seven® (HL7®) permits an interface to be written between a PMS and a billing system, if both have complied with the specifications of the standard. However, if one system is not HL7 compliant, it is much more difficult, if not impossible, to exchange data between the systems. For example, if the dictation system is not HL7 compliant, it will not be able to electronically receive demographic data on patients from the PMS. Another interoperability standard that may be familiar to practices is the Accredited Standards Committee (ASC) X12N standard required under HIPAA for electronic submission of claims and other administrative and financial transactions between providers and payers. Eventually, HIPAA will require electronic claims attachments, which will very likely be HL7-formatted messages contained within an ASC X12N protocol for transmission purposes. This would mean that claims requiring additional information to be sent to the payer would no longer have to be dropped to paper. Retail pharmacies use another standard for transmitting claims and eligibility information. This standard is the National Council for Prescription Drug Programs (NCPDP) Telecommunications Standard. NCPDP also has a SCRIPT standard for use in electronic transmission of prescriptions that providers may find themselves using for electronic prescribing. ASTM International is another standards organization that, in conjunction with several medical specialty societies, has developed a guideline for the content of a continuity of care record (CCR). This standard content is used in conjunction with an HL7 standard for the actual exchange of the data content with referring providers. Refer to Chapter 9, The EHR Regulatory and Standards Environment, for more information on these programs and organizations.

▶ *Comparability standards* are those that ensure consistency of meaning for terms. Sometimes these are called vocabularies, terminologies or code sets. Although slight differences exist among vocabularies, terminologies and code sets, each provides a set of standard terms so there is no misunderstanding among users of systems containing those terms. The most comprehensive and robust medical vocabulary is the Systematized Nomenclature of Medicine, Clinical Terms (SNOMED CT®), developed by the College of American Pathologists (CAP). The National Library of Medicine (NLM) has acquired a license to distribute a version of SNOMED to users free-of-charge. SNOMED, including its microglossaries for nursing terminology and other specialty terms, includes virtually every medical term and defines the relationships among terms. Hence, it is invaluable in creating clinical data repositories. Some EHR vendors have developed proprietary data dictionaries to serve this purpose; but many are migrating to SNOMED as a universal standard. Other terminologies and code sets familiar to practices include the AMA's Current Procedural Terminology (CPT®) and the International Classification of Diseases (ICD). These tend to group concepts and therefore are not as specific as SNOMED. They are used to classify payment information and data for public health purposes. Some experts believe that someday all data in an EHR will be encoded in SNOMED for clinical use as part of structured data entry, and then automatically mapped by the computer to ICD and CPT for billing purposes.

Network and Technical Infrastructure Description

The technology needed to support the EHR components should be described. Once again, first identify everything you have today. If you do not have a network, or have only a very small local area network (LAN), you should still list all devices and components in as much detail as possible. Some of the components you currently have may need to be replaced or upgraded, but there may be a basic infrastructure upon which to build. As you consider subsequent phases, you may not want to specify a network operating system, but consider the exercise the same as for evaluating the database management system (DBMS). You will, however, want to consider the overall structure of your network when you want to extend the network beyond one site, when you want intranet capability (such as for a provider or patient portal), or if and when you want wireless network capability. Other considerations would include special storage capability, additional servers, and scanners (for either a document imaging system or simply to capture limited paper documents electronically). See Chapter 2, EHR Technology, for a more comprehensive description of network and technical infrastructure components.

User Interface Description

HCIs could be included in the network and other technical infrastructure description, but are generally considered so important for user adoption that they are often separately described. HCI technology is described in Chapter 2, EHR Technology, which outlines several options to consider in your decisions with respect to user interfaces. It may be helpful to identify the number of devices currently in place and planned, especially when using the migration path to help you determine costs and benefits for calculating the ROI. The number of devices needed may vary, however, depending on the nature of components being installed. A good guideline is to consider the need for three to four workstations per provider. This equates to one workstation for every provider and associated staff member. In addition, you may want to allocate extra workstations for backup. For special types of user interface devices (e.g., PDA, tablet PC), one per professional with some spares is usually adequate. You should never skimp on user interfaces, as they are key to gaining adoption, and hence benefits realization. Other user interfaces might include printers and scanners (if not included in the technical infrastructure description). Every practice will need printing capability, but the goal of most groups in acquiring an EHR is to achieve a paperless state. In this case, a few high-quality printers may be more appropriate than many small printers.

Operations Description

Operations are described last, but they are by no means the least important. These are the people, policies, and processes needed to make the EHR components work. Identify staffing, key points at which policies change, and other preparatory steps. Many practices underestimate the level of change an EHR introduces. Some are tempted to customize the EHR so that it reflects the existing manual processes. Most changes brought about by IS deployment contribute to improved care and safety, as well as productivity and satisfaction. Practices should be as open as possible to the work flow and process changes suggested by their EHRs.

▶ Conclusion

An EHR is a major investment, certainly equivalent to any medical device acquisition, growth and expansion decision, or building addition. Compared to these latter investments, however, an EHR is a relative unknown.

It directly impacts every person in the practice, and it imposes change where old ways are familiar. Something that has not been directly mentioned yet in this book, but must be considered, is the dynamic nature of the EHR marketplace. EHR components have many options. Many vendors have entered – and left – the market. The volatility of the market is a concern, but as it is settling down, better products remain and emerge. Finally, the risk-reward equation is great. There is great risk in making the right choice, but the reward can be huge if the EHR is fully adopted and deployed.

NOTES

1. eHealth Initiative, "Electronic Prescribing: Toward Maximum Value and Rapid Adoption," Washington, DC: eHealth Initiative, April 14, 2004 (www.ehealthinitiative.org/initiatives/erx/).
2. Council for Affordable Quality Healthcare (CAQH), "Promoting Interoperability: Online Eligibility and Benefits Inquiry," September 13, 2004 (www.caqh.org/press_caqh_press.html).
3. Margret\A Consulting, LLC, "HIPAA Transactions and Code Sets Toolkit for Physicians and Other Providers of Professional Healthcare Services," distributed by Blue Cross and Blue Shield Association.
4. Phase II Stark Regulations Interim Final Rule (69 Federal Register 16054), effective July 26, 2004.

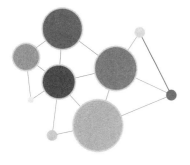

▶ FOUR

Return on Investment

Most practices want to determine a return on investment (ROI) for their particular EHR system. This will help them determine the financial feasibility of acquiring the type of system they have in mind. ROI analysis should also help practices benchmark the benefits they get from their EHR once it is implemented to make sure they are realizing the expected benefits.

In simplest terms, ROI is the calculation of when the financial value of the benefits meets the cost of the system. This is when the practice knows it has "paid for" the system – known as the payback period. Other more sophisticated ROI measures, such as internal rate of return, may also be determined.

As described in Chapter 1, Introduction and Rationale for EHRs, EHR systems offer many types of benefits. Chapter 2, EHR Technology, outlines the types of technology that typically are used in an EHR implementation. Chapter 3, Determining Your Group's Objectives, describes a migration path for which benefits increase with the greater sophistication of systems. This chapter provides tools to measure these benefits and determine the cost of the type of system being considered. In addition, it shows how to analyze this information.

Some practices leave ROI analysis up to the vendor. Although vendor ROI can be very helpful because vendors know their products and have seen them in action in other practices, be aware that vendors will necessarily want to paint a rosy picture. It behooves every practice to make its own estimates first, and then adjust the estimates based on factors learned from the vendor, references, and other research.

THIS CHAPTER ASSISTS in the ROI process by helping you:

- ▶ Quantify benefits from EHR systems;
- ▶ Identify and develop financial benefits assumptions;
- ▶ Identify costs of EHR systems;
- ▶ Calculate the ROI payback period for an EHR system;
- ▶ Understand other ROI measures; and
- ▶ Appreciate the value of a benefits realization activity.

▶ EHR Benefits

Chapter 1, Introduction and Rationale for EHRs, shows that although benefits are clearly achievable from EHR systems, they are not easy to quantify, let alone translate into financial terms. However, the more specific you can be about the nature of the technology and applications you plan to acquire, the more likely you will be able to produce a realistic estimate of ROI.

As discussed in Chapter 1, Introduction and Rationale for EHRs, EHRs have quantifiable benefits vs. anecdotal benefits, as well as financial benefits vs. qualitative benefits. It is important to distinguish among these and to ensure that your ROI calculations do not estimate financial benefits that are unrealistic. For example, a common tactic by vendors is to add up all the time saved through increased productivity, determine the value of that time at the average salary and benefits rates for the respective staff members, and present the result as a cost savings. There are definitely productivity improvements from EHR systems, and some may result in staff reductions, but most such productivity improvements only allow staff to do a better job and direct more of their attention to patients and patient care. It is certainly rare that a 0.2 full-time equivalent (FTE) of a nurse will be eliminated from the practice, even though the time saved with the EHR may represent 0.2 FTE. Exhibit 4.1 provides examples of each type of benefit.

EXHIBIT 4.1	**Types of Benefits** 101101001010010100100001000110011001000110001	
Quality	Reduction in medication errors by 70%	Provider satisfaction that a diagnosis for a patient was not missed
Financial	$3,000 was saved in transcription cost	Nursing staff have more time for patient instruction
	Quantifiable	**Anecdotal**

▶ Benefits Portfolio

The mix of financial, qualitative, quantifiable, and anecdotal benefits may be considered a benefits portfolio. The value of the entire portfolio is important, even though only those benefits that can be quantified in financial terms will be used in calculating ROI.

Constructing a benefits portfolio can also help determine if there are ways to estimate the financial value of some of the qualitative and anecdotal benefits. Be aware, however, that financial value can be used in an ROI calculation only where it has a direct financial impact on the practice. The scenario in Exhibit 4.2 on the next page is an example of the complexity involved.

A good way to document a benefits portfolio is illustrated in Exhibit 4.3 on pages 87–88. The purpose of documenting such a portfolio is to ensure that all members of the practice recognize the full value of the EHR. This helps set expectations for achieving these benefits.

In documenting the benefits portfolio, identify benefits as quantifiable metrics if possible. Quantification helps in reaching agreement on the importance and helps ensure awareness of whether the benefit is being accomplished. Link the specific metrics for the benefit to the source of the benefit in the EHR. If, for some reason, the benefit is not achieved by the time frame anticipated, there may be problems with the intended source.

Because of the complexity and variety of benefits in a benefits portfolio that are not necessarily financial, most practices tend to look for financial benefits through operational improvements from their EHRs. Such benefits include those identified in Exhibit 4.4 on page 88.

EXHIBIT 4.2 Complexity of Benefits Determination 00010001100

Reduction in medication errors is very important. Some of the benefits may be described as:

1. Ensuring that patients do not get sicker or die on the medications they have been prescribed, making for healthier and happier patients;

2. Less likelihood that patients will file a malpractice suit due to medication errors;

3. Less expenditure the health plan has to make for additional care due to medication errors;

4. Potentially lower insurance premiums for the patient or patient's sponsor (employer, Medicare, Medicaid) if there are fewer medication errors; or

5. A stronger economy as a result of happier and healthier patients who can be at work and productive.

However, not all of these benefits directly translate into reduced costs or increased revenue for the provider. Those that may contribute to reduced costs or increased revenue include:

▶ Being able to demonstrate a low medication error rate may mean a favorable position with respect to contract negotiation. You may be able to negotiate a lower required discount for discounted fee-for-service patients or a larger proportion of fees retained in a managed care contract. A practice considering acquiring an EHR should contact its major payers to determine if these or other such pay-for-performance (P4P) incentives are viable and what requirements are necessary for documentation.

▶ Lessening the likelihood of malpractice suits can also potentially reduce malpractice premiums for the provider. Again, contact the insurer to determine how the acquisition of an EHR may impact these costs.

▶ Increasing the patient base, and therefore revenue, represent a benefit. It is conceivable that quality indicators made possible through an EHR, if made public in a community, may draw patients to the practice. In the absence of such public accountability (as is increasingly called for in hospitals, and potentially soon for providers), patients may judge for themselves that "wired" providers are better providers. Even though this may increasingly be a factor in patient choice, however, few research studies support specific measures. Being "wired" can also be part of a practice's advertising strategy to entice new patients.

Reprinted with permission, Margret\A Consulting, LLC

EXHIBIT 4.3 Benefits Portfolio 0110100101001010010000010001100

EXPECTED BENEFITS	METRICS	SOURCE	TIME FRAME
1. Data availability	1.1 Charts available to all users when needed	1.1 Document imaging	March Yr. 1
	1.2 Results available to all users when needed	1.2 Results fed directly from computer output into the document management system (COLD feed)	June Yr. 1
	1.3	1.3	
2. Provider productivity	2.1 All providers will leave office at designated time	2.1 Work flow tools	June Yr. 1
	2.2 Calls from pharmacies about new prescriptions will be reduced by 60%	2.2 E-prescribing tools	September Yr. 1
	2.3 Calls from pharmacies about refills will be reduced by 80%	2.3 E-prescribing tools	June Yr. 1
	2.4	2.4	
3. Service efficiency	3.1 No patients will need to be rescheduled for missing results	3.1 Document management system	June Yr. 1
	3.2	3.2	
4. Operational savings	4.1 Chart pulls will be reduced by 30%	4.1 Document management system	June Yr. 1
	4.2 Chart pulls will be reduced by 60%	4.1 Document management system and abstraction	December Yr. 1
	4.3	4.3	
5. Data quality	5.1		
6. Patient satisfaction	6.1	6.1	
7. Service quality	7.1	7.1	
8. Patient safety	8.1	8.1	

continued next page

EXHIBIT 4.3 Benefits Portfolio *continued* 0100101001000010001100

EXPECTED BENEFITS	METRICS	SOURCE	TIME FRAME
9. Patient outcomes	9.1	9.1	
10. Cost of care	10.1	10.1	
11. Quality of life	11.1	11.1	
12. Population health	12.1	12.1	

Reprinted with permission, Margret\A Consulting, LLC

Within each type of benefit are many specific examples. What financial benefits you will actually get from your EHR depends on the type of EHR you implement (see the EHR benefits matrix, Exhibit 3.1 in Chapter 3, Determining Your Group's Objectives) and the extent to which it is truly adopted by all in the practice.

EXHIBIT 4.4 Types of Financial Benefits 1001010010000010001100

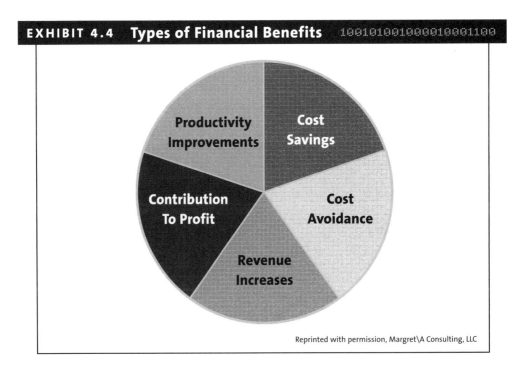

Reprinted with permission, Margret\A Consulting, LLC

Productivity Improvements

Productivity improvements may lead to direct cost savings. Some productivity improvements that lead to direct cost savings include:

▶ *Reduced overtime costs for staff.* If the EHR supports work flow changes and process improvements, staff members who frequently do not complete their assigned duties in the time allotted due to, for example, constant interruptions from telephone calls, missing charts, misfiled documents, or re-work will find these time-wasters have gone away. Even though most practices have found real reductions in this area, they manage reduced overtime carefully because some staff depend on the extra income and may not be amenable to making the necessary work flow changes to eliminate overtime.

▶ *Elimination of outsourcing expenses.* Many providers use billing services to help with coding, billing, accounts receivable management, and collections. If the EHR supports coding as the provider is documenting in the system, external coding resources may not be needed on a full-time basis (although they probably will continue to be needed for auditing). EHRs that are interfaced or integrated with a practice management system (PMS) and make full use of the various administrative and financial transactions with health plans can lead to a reduction in the need for billing support, accounts receivable management, and collections. The practice may possibly bring those functions in-house and re-deploy staff who faced elimination through other productivity gains.

▶ *Additional patient time.* If only data access functionality is supported by the system, productivity gains may be modest. If documentation is actually performed on the EHR, however, more significant gains may be achieved. Although some providers may perceive that it takes longer to enter data into an EHR, the downstream productivity savings from improved work flows and process improvements are sufficiently great enough that some practices have found a 10 to 15 percent increase in the number of patients seen in a day, according to one study.[1] Another study found that office visit time was reduced by 13 percent for physicians because of faster pre-encounter chart review and post-encounter recording of data in the chart, although physician's time with the patients stayed the same.[2]

▶ *Fractional FTE savings.* Although real, fractional FTE savings generally do not represent actual financial cost savings. Some productivity improvements are actually more qualitative than financial. For example, although evidence exists that nurse productivity is improved by reducing the number of telephone calls that must be handled, or reducing nurse intake and chart documentation time (in one study by 15 minutes for new visits and 20 minutes for return visits[3]), this will not necessarily eliminate nursing time. Instead, the nurse will use the time for better patient care. However, if your practice has a difficult time with nurse retention, there may be cost savings associated with nurse recruitment if the nurses are happier using an EHR and willing to remain on the job (which is actually being demonstrated in some hospital environments).[4] EHRs are also found to be an attractive incentive to join a practice.

Cost Savings

Cost savings may accrue from a variety of sources:

▶ *Eliminating paper chart supplies.* If document imaging is deployed or if the EHR supports full clinician documentation and the contents of the EHR are not routinely printed and filed, there can be significant savings in the costs of forms printing, folders, and fax and printer supplies. Such supplies cost an estimated $3 per chart.[5] In addition, the costs of paper storage, such as the need for microfilming or storing charts in a warehouse, can be reduced. Transportation costs for internal staff or courier services can also be eliminated if charts must be delivered to different locations. These costs include not only personnel time, but the depreciation cost of the vehicles, insurance, maintenance, and upkeep. Costs of creating printouts from the EHR, however, must be monitored closely. This cost savings will not accrue if clinicians routinely print copies only for the purpose of reading a chart, which should be done online.

▶ *Reducing clerical personnel.* If an EHR is acquired, documentation is supported, and all clinicians agree to document in the EHR, some clerical staff positions can possibly be eliminated. (At one large clinic, after EHR implementation, the cost of chart pulls went from $20 per chart pulled to less than $1 per chart pulled because there were so few charts pulled.[6] This is an unusual case – both in the original cost as well as the striking improvement.) In most cases, however, some clerical staff must be retained for scanning documents that come to the practice in paper form and for various printing activities. In fact, if your practice chooses to use document imaging as its form of EHR, staff pulling and filing paper charts will be redeployed to scanning paper and there will generally be no cost savings. Furthermore, if not all clinicians document via the EHR or if the EHR includes only certain components of the record, and other components must be retained on paper, the cost of managing parallel medical record systems or hybrid medical record systems can be higher than the cost of managing paper systems alone.

▶ *Reducing transcription costs.* Cost savings may also accrue by reducing the amount of transcription, whether using in-house transcriptionists or a service. If the EHR will be used for documentation by the clinician at the point of care, a significant amount of transcription costs can be eliminated. Such transcription savings can be from $300 to more than $1,000 per month per physician.[7] Further transcription cost reduction can be achieved if the EHR can create patient summaries and if it will contribute to a continuity of care record (CCR). The actual savings, of course, depends on the amount currently being spent on transcription. (Note that if there is concern about redeploying transcriptionists, they may be used as correctionists if speech dictation is employed, or the practice may find it feasible to sell transcription services to other providers and realize new transcription revenue.

▶ *Eliminating copy service.* Many practices use a copy service to respond to requests for information from attorneys, insurance companies, and other providers. The cost of the copy service can be saved if documents can be printed from the EHR in the practice. There will be even more savings if other providers and patients are given limited access to information through a provider/patient portal, or if a CCR and personal health record (PHR) are generated. For example, through automation, turnaround time for referrals was reportedly reduced from one day to less than one hour.[8] Furthermore, if claims attachments are sent electronically to payers, this copying cost is also eliminated.

▶ *Eliminating generation of paperwork to patients.* Statements and other paper notices to patients can be reduced, if not eliminated. If eligibility verification and co-pay collections are performed, it is possible to eliminate the generation of patient statements and their associated mailing costs. Although this is not necessarily a function of an EHR (i.e., it is more a function of a PMS), most practices will not adopt such electronic transaction processing until they start using more advanced computer systems, such as EHRs. It is also possible to eliminate generation of paper notices of privacy practices, patient instructions, and other materials if patients are directed to the practice's Web site or kiosk in the office.

▶ *Reducing collection fees.* The cost of a collection system can also be reduced if eligibility verification and collection of co-pays are performed at the time of the visit.

▶ *Reducing malpractice premiums.* Cost savings associated with reduced malpractice premiums through the use of EHRs would be included in this category. Check with your malpractice insurance carrier to see whether it offers this advantage and if so, what percentage may be reduced. This might even be the right time to look at other carriers in your area to investigate other options.

Cost Avoidance

Cost avoidance means the office will not have to incur an anticipated cost. For example, if you are running out of storage space, an EHR will help you avoid the costs of storing the records in a warehouse or microfilming them. (Note that this is a cost savings if you incur the cost now and can eliminate it. It is cost avoidance if the cost is not incurred now but will have to be during the period of time you are acquiring the EHR.) If your EHR includes a patient portal by which patients can make their own appointments and get educational information, you may not have to hire an additional telephone receptionist as patient volume increases. The cost of additional space might be avoided if the practice plans to add another provider and can turn a file room into the needed space.

Revenue Increases

Revenue increases from an EHR are very real:

▶ *Improved documentation.* Improved documentation yields significant revenue increases. This is due to the Evaluation and Management (E&M) coding support embedded in many EHR systems, as well as to the use of practice guidelines that provide for more complete documentation. Revenue increases due to improved documentation for coding are reported to be between 3 and 15 percent.[9] EHR automatic generation and transmission of charges to the billing system can reduce the number of lost charges and days in accounts receivable (A/R days).[10] Fully captured revenue from inpatient care can also be improved, especially if the provider carries a wireless personal digital assistant (PDA) that uploads data upon entering the office.

► *Contract negotiation.* Revenue increases can be achieved by being in a better position to negotiate managed care contracts because you have better data on your outcomes, you can demonstrate fewer medication errors, and you can document closer adherence to a health plan's formulary. More favorable discounts in discounted fee-for-service environments are feasible. Different P4P models are also on the horizon and should be negotiable based on improved patient care through the use of an EHR.

► *Added time to see more patients.* The additional patient revenue is real; however, do not count this financial benefit twice if it is already identified under improved productivity. A more realistic revenue source may be increased revenue by increasing the number of services. Some EHR systems provide the practice with support for searching records for overdue services, such as immunizations, health screenings and tests, and they automatically send reminder notices to patients. E-prescribing systems that provide fill status notification can alert you when a patient has not completed a medication regimen, potentially warranting a visit.

► *Participation in clinical trials.* Because an EHR can assist your practice to identify candidates for clinical trials, your ability to participate in clinical trials will increase, which can generate revenue.

► *Selling new services.* Transcription services have already been mentioned. Other potential services center around the EHR itself. Some practices are providing data center hosting services for others, and some physicians and administrators, having gone through the process of integrating a system, teach others by offering EHR consulting services. Sometimes having the ability to electronically manage an inventory, for example, can lead to extended product offerings through the practice, such as herbal supplements, special cosmetics, clothing (e.g., mastectomy bras or exercise wear), or other devices, such as foot care products.

Contribution to Profit

Contribution to profit is achieved primarily through the combination of productivity improvements and revenue increases because you are able to keep more of the revenue you earn. However, especially in a managed-care situation, the following are potential ways to contribute to profit:

► Avoiding repeat diagnostic tests;

► Using less expensive medications; and

► Making appropriate referrals.

Other Financial Benefits

Although a number of other benefits accrue from EHRs, such as more complete and legible documentation, built-in reminders and alerts, in-basket functionality for interoffice communications, electronic signature capability, and remote connectivity, be very careful to not overestimate the financial value of such benefits. If you cannot actually see where a true dollar savings or new revenue will result, do not include it in your benefits calculations. It is important to recognize and appreciate these other benefits of EHRs, but they should not be factored into ROI calculations.

Use the benefits worksheet in Exhibit 4.5 to capture your financial benefits data. Phase in benefits over the period of time that reflects your implementation and adoption cycle, as well your migration path. For example, if you plan to implement clinical messaging as a first phase, and to delay implementing documentation and decision support for three years, you should not estimate cost savings from reduction in paper chart supplies or clerical services until the start of the second phase of your EHR implementation. As another example, if you anticipate that only 20 percent of providers will document directly into the EHR in the first year, reduce these costs by only 20 percent in the first year. (These examples are shown in italics on Exhibit 4.5).

You should segregate each project phase for purposes of comparing with costs. This can readily be done by explicitly identifying the actual years for which benefits data are being estimated.

Benefits Worksheet

As you use the benefits worksheet, be sure to document the types of benefits assumptions you make. You may need to reference these assumptions as you present your ROI analysis to those who will make the ultimate decision about the investment. They may challenge the assumptions, want to be more conservative, or decide to be more directive and require adoption of the EHR such that the assumptions can be more aggressive. You can record your assumptions directly on the financial benefits worksheet, as shown in Exhibit 4.5, or you can record them in a separate document. Just be sure they are readily available for review of the analysis. In addition, you may need to refer to them during contract negotiations. You may find that vendors are willing to provide vendor discounts if their particular product meets reasonable ROI expectations. You may also want to keep your assumptions to help you determine whether expected benefits for the practice are

EXHIBIT 4.5 Benefits Worksheet 101001010010100100001000110

BENEFITS	CURRENT COSTS	MIGRATION PATH PHASES 1 AND 2			MIGRATION PATH PHASES 3 AND 4	
		YEAR__	YEAR__	YEAR__	YEAR__	YEAR__
Overtime reduction						
Assumptions:						
Outsourcing reduction						
Assumptions:						
Other productivity						
Assumptions:						
Paper chart supplies					$1,000	$3,900
Assumptions:					*20% of $2.50/ chart for 2,000 charts*	*60% of $2.60/ chart for 2,500 charts*
Clerical chart costs	$22,400					$25,160
Assumptions (clerk time):						0.5 FTE @ $23,500 + 12% = $13,160
Assumptions (courier costs):						$25/run twice/day 240 days/ yr. = $12,000
Transcription costs						
Assumptions:						
Copy service costs						
Assumptions:						
Paper statement costs						
Assumptions:						
Malpractice premiums						
Assumptions:						
Storage costs						
Assumptions:						
Archival space costs						
Assumptions:						

continued next page

EXHIBIT 4.5 **Benefits Worksheet** *continued* 0010100100000100001100

BENEFITS	CURRENT COSTS	MIGRATION PATH PHASES 1 AND 2			MIGRATION PATH PHASES 3 AND 4	
		YEAR__	YEAR__	YEAR__	YEAR__	YEAR__
Additional staff costs						
Assumptions:						
Coding improvements						
Assumptions:						
Lost charges						
Assumptions:						
Penalties/Denials						
Assumptions						
Discounts/Incentives						
Assumptions:						
New service revenue						
Assumptions:						
Clinical trials revenue						
Assumptions:						
Avoidance of tests						
Assumptions:						
Medication costs						
Assumptions:						
Referrals						
Assumptions:						
Assumptions:						
Assumptions:						
TOTAL BENEFITS						

Reprinted with permission, Margret\A Consulting, LLC

being met. You may not have to do a formal benefits realization study, but you may find it helpful to compare your anticipated savings with actual savings to take corrective action if expectations are not being met.

As you develop your calculations, be sure to include all associated costs and increases expected over time. For example, if your practice currently pays clerical staff a $20,000 salary per year plus 12 percent benefits, the fully loaded cost of a clerk is $22,400 ($20,000 x 1.12). If you don't anticipate realizing clerical cost savings for five years, however, you need to anticipate cost-of-living or performance increases over time. The example in Exhibit 4.5 uses an estimate of $23,500 for the future salary.

Also be sure, as you estimate your costs and potential savings, to use actual data from your practice. For example, the average cost of paper chart supplies was estimated earlier to be $3 per chart. Your actual cost, however, may be different. Exhibit 4.5 uses costs of $2.50 for the first year and $2.60 for the second year of the EHR because they represent actual costs for the sample practice. Note that this sample practice also plans an increase in the number of new patients, so the number of charts being created would increase as well.

Finally, as you use the benefits worksheet in Exhibit 4.5, feel free to add or delete potential benefit categories to fit your practice. If you find that many of the categories of benefits might not apply to your practice, however, you may want to retain the categories to demonstrate that more sophisticated systems or better adoption rates would yield more benefits.

▶ Costs of EHR Systems

Once financial benefits of EHR systems are estimated, you must turn your attention to calculating total costs of the EHR. Some experts suggest calculating costs prior to benefits to avoid a bias that could result in skimping on costs. The alternative could also be true, however – calculating costs prior to benefits could introduce a bias in being less conservative in savings estimates. Suffice it to say that both exercises must be done without bias. Once total benefits and total costs for the desired system are identified, go back and see how adjustments can be made.

Just as there are categories of financial benefits, there are categories of financial costs. Some experts attempt to ascribe proportions to these costs, but this will vary by what the practice already has and can capitalize on, what resources are available for support, the type of EHR system acquired, as well as many other factors. Exhibit 4.6 shown on the next page summarizes the types of financial costs for an EHR system.

EXHIBIT 4.6   Types of Financial Costs 0010100101001000010001100

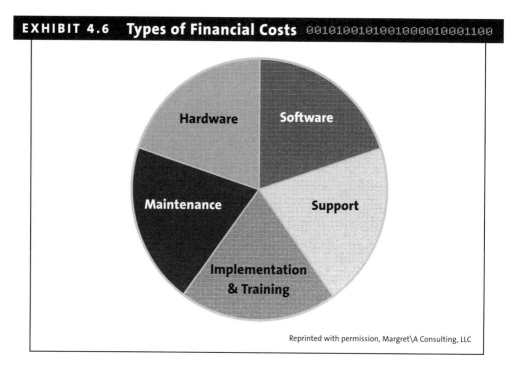

Reprinted with permission, Margret\A Consulting, LLC

In addition to types of costs, there are also initial, or first year, costs and ongoing, or annual, costs. It is generally advisable to do a cost estimate for at least the first year plus two to four additional years.

Hardware

Hardware costs consist of computer equipment as well as network devices. The cost of servers may be among the largest single costs, unless the practice already has made an investment or plans to enter into a time-sharing agreement with another source that has purchased the servers. As noted in Chapter 2, EHR Technology, this is not the place for cost cutting.

A robust server(s) or server services are essential to user adoption of an EHR. If the system appears slow, users will become very frustrated, and there is a good chance they will not use the system. A server for a small- to medium-sized practice may cost in the area of $5,000 to $15,000. It is also critical to have not only the main server but also a backup server or at least backup server capability. Because an EHR becomes a mission-critical element in the practice, full redundancy is essential. The redundant server is carrying the exact same load as the main server, so its cost is essentially the same.

Hardware costs for backup and storage will also need to include data storage media, such as redundant array of inexpensive disk (RAID) arrays and tape cartridges, as well as various drives to process the storage media. Your EHR vendor or disaster recovery vendor should be able to advise you on the nature of the backup hardware needed and what price range that represents. Be sure to budget annually for replacement of data storage media because disks and tapes may need replacement or additions to accommodate more data.

Human-computer interfaces (HCIs), or input devices, are also critical hardware. HCIs must be ubiquitous. Every office, exam room, registration area, conference room, and other practice area needs to be considered. Prior to the advent of portable, wireless devices, practices estimated the need at between three and six computers per provider, at a cost of about $1,500 per computer. Some practices, however, are finding that savings measures can be taken by adopting portable, wireless devices that the providers can take with them as they move from office to exam room, conference room, or remote areas. This is a significant work flow change, however, so it needs to be assessed carefully before making any decisions. Also, in some cases, the unit cost of these devices is actually higher than a typical PC, although fewer of them may be needed. Notebook and tablet computers can cost close to $2,000; whereas PDAs may cost $500 to $750. Note that your local computer store may sell cheaper devices, but ensure that the quality of screen, size of random access memory (RAM), and other features are sufficient for continual use throughout a day and beyond.

Even though the number of devices per provider may be reduced with portable, wireless devices, having spare devices is important if the portable device gets left at home or at the hospital or while it is charging. Remember also that one size does not fit all. Some providers may prefer tablets over PDAs, or prefer notebooks in the exam room and tablets for remote connectivity in the office or conference room.

HCIs (and for that matter, all types of hardware) are very dynamic. Significantly new devices are created every 12 to 18 months. Although everyone doesn't need the latest and greatest all the time, there are benefits to budgeting for an obsolescence factor. (Considering that many people buy new cars every three years, you have an idea of how dynamic the computer market is.)

Other input devices must also be included. Even if an office is not planning to use document imaging as its primary means of acquiring an EHR, at least one scanner should be available to scan external records and certain documents. A single scanner may cost a few hundred dollars. However, if document imaging is performed, much higher quality imaging systems are needed, and these can cost several thousand dollars each. If speech recognition is chosen, microphone capability must be purchased. If there is interest in patient access to information, one or more kiosks containing computers, or at least monitors, may be needed. (Frequently, only touch-screen monitors are used and connected via the network to the server.)

Printers, faxes, and other output devices are included in hardware costs, even though their numbers should be moderate in comparison to the input devices. Remember, the ideal is to perform all functions electronically, not via paper. Still, even the most paperless office will need a printer for release of information, response to subpoenas, and other uses. Depending on the nature of the printer, this can run from several hundred to a thousand or more dollars.

Network devices, such as routers, switches, wireless access points, and so forth, are all part of network hardware expenditures. Telecommunication devices, such as modems, multiplexers, cable, and so forth, may be sold as part of a telecommunication package purchased with telecommunication services, or may have to be purchased separately. The size and topology of the network determines the devices, so it is possible to provide only an estimated range: All network components for a small office should cost between $5,000 and $10,000.

Electrical equipment should also be considered in hardware costs. Uninterruptible power supplies, costing a few hundred dollars each, are critical. Some offices may even consider acquiring a backup generator.

Another type of hardware cost that is sometimes overlooked is that of new cabinets and other furniture that may be needed to house computer equipment. This may include remodeling some space for a "data center," building a shelf in each exam room onto which to a rest a tablet PC while examining a patient, buying a printer stand, using a kiosk, creating a well in the registration desk so there is still workspace on the desk, and many other "low tech" or "no tech" elements.

Software

Software generally means licenses for the operating system and the applications themselves, as well as the cost of interfaces.

Operating system software may come packaged with the hardware devices. If licensed separately, you must determine what operating system software is needed per device. Server operating system software is often different than client operating system software. Here again, the software depends upon the EHR purchased. Operating system software, however, is generally a relatively small proportion of the overall cost of software.

Application software is the major software expense. Vendors price software licenses in a variety of ways – per physician, per site, per workstation, or per "user," among others. The vendor has the most latitude for giving a vendor discount on application software. But be aware that the vendor that is willing to deeply discount the application software will likely make up the difference in implementation costs and/or maintenance fees, or may be less willing to bundle subscription service expenses into the package. In addition, be sure that you have the right number of licenses because that will impact the validity of your license and maintenance agreements. Application software for a comprehensive EHR providing documentation and clinical decision support can easily range between $5,000 and $25,000. Although this is a very wide range, the old adage "you get what you pay for" truly applies.

The above description of application software assumes only one package for an EHR. Many EHRs, however, comprise modules; for example, there may be a basic messaging module, document-imaging module, documentation module, clinical decision support module, e-prescribing module, PHR module, and so forth. Another possibility is that there is one package with a few complementary modules, such as report writers, speech recognition, etc. As noted above, it is critical to understand what is being purchased and how it is being packaged – both to obtain accurate cost data and to ensure that you are acquiring a complete system.

One factor many practices forget to consider in licensing application software is the potential need to upgrade other existing applications. For example, you may have a PMS that was last upgraded for Health Insurance Portability and Accountability Act of 1996 (HIPAA) transactions a few years ago. A newer version may be available, but you just haven't acquired it. To link the EHR to the PMS, however, you may have to acquire the latest version or at least a certain newer version.

You must also consider interfaces if you are linking your EHR to your PMS or any other information system. Be aware that even if systems come from the same vendor you may still need an interface. Generally, this is a less costly, easier, and more successful interface than if there were different vendors, but the additional cost may be still be substantial. If you have different systems, you will have to consider interfaces. Unfortunately, if the existing systems are not HL7 compatible or the vendor has gone out of business, attempting to get an interface written could actually be more costly than acquiring the fully integrated product from the EHR vendor. Remember also that an interface is often two pieces of software: one from the new EHR to the old system and one from the old system to the new EHR system. A single interface may cost a few thousand dollars or more.

In addition to the operating system and EHR application, along with upgrades, interfaces, or replacement modules, practices may also be looking at acquiring Microsoft Office® software, project management software, and backup software, as well as special software for other purposes. All of these costs must be included in the cost estimate. Some practices are even looking into acquiring rights to the source code for the EHR applications, and there may be a separate fee for that.

Support

"Support" may mean different things to different people. In this context, it means all the elements associated with planning for and selecting the EHR, conducting special implementation activities, and providing ongoing user support.

In some cases, practices will not add these costs to the cost worksheet, instead considering them a part of normal operations. Whether any or all of these costs are included in the ROI calculations for EHR acquisition is a matter of practice policy.

Support costs may include:

▶ A consultant to help with EHR readiness assessment, vendor selection, and contract negotiation;

▶ Travel costs to attend trade shows and/or conduct site visits to learn more about EHRs;

▶ Subscriptions to publications to acquire special research on EHR systems;

▶ Cost of accreditation – a very new activity that is just being developed, often by special associations or other organizations, but which may impact your ability to get cost incentives for using the EHR (these may be one-time or ongoing costs);

▶ Physician compensation to conduct quality improvement projects associated with use of the EHR and to continually build and maintain clinical practice guidelines and structured data templates, as well as to refine clinical decision support (CDS); this cost may be a few hours a week for a small practice to virtually full time for a very large practice); or

▶ Contract costs with the EHR vendor, consultant, or other specialty vendor to provide ongoing hardware and software maintenance – this might be a remote help desk or network and/or systems analyst who performs routine maintenance.

Contingency planning is especially important with such a mission-critical system as an EHR, and especially in certain regions of the country. Contingency planning can take various forms. Emergency mode operation and disaster recovery service fees may include the development of an emergency mode operation plan and/or disaster recovery plan. It may also include a subscription to a special site that is maintained in preparation for assisting the provider in the event of an emergency or disaster. These are sometimes graded by the degree to which the site is "ready" for use: A hot site may be a fully replicated version of your data center; a warm site may be a facility that provides basic utility services and general-purpose computers; a cold site may simply be warehouse space in a distant location. Another alternative is a reciprocal site where several providers or providers with other businesses – such as schools, local fire departments, or others – agree to host each other in the event of an emergency or disaster.

Implementation and Training

Implementation and training costs are generally one-time costs directly associated with adopting the EHR. They include:

▶ Vendor fees for implementation support, including travel to your location(s);

▶ Training fees and travel expenses for special training offered by the vendor;

▶ Upgrading the pay of one of the staff members to be a project manager (or hiring relief staff to free a person part time for being a project manager);

▶ Compensating physicians for loss of revenue during the time they are engaging in planning for and learning the system;

▶ Overtime pay for staff to be trained;

▶ Attorney fees to review the vendor contract;

▶ Cost of an electrician to do wiring;

▶ Contractor costs to build special cabinets, etc.;

▶ Cost of engaging a network and/or systems analyst consultant to work side-by-side with the vendor to install the system;

▶ Fees for temporary staff or an outsourcing company to convert data from one system to another, to abstract data from paper charts into the EHR, or to scan documents from paper charts into a repository; and

▶ Engaging a webmaster to develop a Web site for the practice.

Maintenance

Maintenance generally refers to all ongoing costs associated with hardware and software.

Hardware maintenance would include the cost of service contracts and/or service calls. It may also include replacement equipment. When budgeting, be sure to discount the first year's maintenance by the amount represented by the warranty period.

Annual software maintenance may cost between 10 and 25 percent of the initial software cost. Maintenance costs include:

▶ Ongoing software license fees;

▶ Any fees associated with maintenance agreements to supply patches and upgrades;

▶ Costs of additional user training;

▶ Subscription fees for access to reference materials and knowledge sources (e.g., subscription to a drug knowledge base);

▶ Vocabulary usage fees;

► Transaction fees for obtaining medication history from pharmacy benefits managers;

► EHR vendor user group fees and/or attendance at meetings;

► Ongoing licenses for patient instructional material or health educational material for a Web site;

► Webmaster services to keep a Web site up to date;

► Telecommunication fees (e.g., Digital Subscriber Line [DSL] or cable services, wireless access services, Internet Provider Services); and

► Potentially many others.

Cost Worksheet

Use a cost worksheet, such as shown in Exhibit 4.7 to plot all potential costs for the EHR. Just as with the benefits worksheet, it is important to document your assumptions. Some of this is built into the worksheet, but other information might be more appropriately filed in separate notes or quotes from vendors.

Once the cost worksheet has been completed, the first step generally is to determine whether there is sufficient capital to even make the investment. Loans or other sources of financing may have to be sought. Pushing back on some of the investment may be necessary. The practice may have to go back to its migration path and cut back on early expenditures while reaping some of the gains that can be reinvested. Obviously, the results should be discussed with the vendor to investigate areas that can be trimmed. Be very cautious, however, in trimming expenses without realizing fewer benefits and potentially greater risk. For example, if you decide not to buy the back-up server, what would be the consequences if the first server failed? Sometimes it's better to put off an investment rather than to cut back so drastically that there is greater potential for problems.

Note that the cost worksheet in Exhibit 4.7 on pages 106–7 is set up to record initial and ongoing costs for *one* project phase. When comparing this with the benefits worksheet in Exhibit 4.5, you will need to specify to which project phase you are estimating costs (if there is only one phase in which you acquire all components of an EHR, you would need only one worksheet). You should also make sure you estimate both benefits and costs for the same number of total years (usually three or five).

EXHIBIT 4.7 Cost Worksheet 010110100101001010010000010001100

COST ELEMENTS FOR PHASE _____ EHR _____	ASSUMPTIONS (ONLY ONE PHASE)	INITIAL UNIT COST	QTY	TOTAL INITIAL COST	ANNUAL COST YR. 1	ANNUAL COST YRS. 2-5	TOTAL ANNUAL COSTS
HARDWARE							
Main server	May be time-shared						
Backup server	May be time-shared						
Other server(s)	Specify purpose(s)						
Storage devices	Describe						
Storage media	Describe						
Input devices	Workstations						
	Other:_____						
Output devices	Printers						
	Other:_____						
Network devices	List						
Telecom devices	List						
Electrical devices	List						
SOFTWARE							
Operating system	Describe license						
EHR package	Describe license						
Modules							
Components							
Upgrades	Identify						
Interfaces	Describe						
Other software	List						
SUPPORT							
Selection consultant	Operations?						
EHR education	Operations?						
Publications	Operations?						
Accreditation	Specify						
MD QI support	Percentage						
Hardware & software support	Fees						
Contingency support	Fees						

EXHIBIT 4.7   Cost Worksheet *continued*   010100101001000010001100

COST ELEMENTS FOR PHASE _EHR_	ASSUMPTIONS (ONLY ONE PHASE)	INITIAL UNIT COST	QTY	TOTAL INITIAL COST	ANNUAL COST YR. 1	ANNUAL COST YRS. 2-5	TOTAL ANNUAL COSTS
IMPLEMENTATION AND TRAINING							
Vendor fees	Negotiated						
Training (incl. travel)	Describe						
Project manager	Percentage						
MD loss of revenue	Amount						
Overtime	Amount						
Attorney	Fees						
Electrician	Fees						
Contractor	Fees						
Implement consultant	Fees						
Data conversion	Fees						
Webmaster	Fees						
MAINTENANCE							
Hardware service	List and describe						
Software licenses	List and describe						
Subscriptions	List						
Telecom fees	Fees						
ISP fees	Fees						
TOTALS							

Reprinted with permission, Margret\A Consulting, LLC

▶ ROI Calculations

Once benefits and costs are estimated, ROI calculations can be made. The first step is to summarize and record costs and benefits. Sample data are provided in the ROI calculation worksheet in Exhibit 4.8. The cost data (estimated here) would come from a cost worksheet (see Exhibit 4.7). The benefits data, which here are conservative estimates for a project that has only one phase of acquiring the EHR, would come from a benefits worksheet such as shown in Exhibit 4.5. The result is a quite typical three-and-a-half-year payback period. Although some vendors estimate far shorter payback periods, such estimates are almost always based on staff productivity improvements that are real, but do not result in staff layoffs and therefore reduced out-of-pocket costs. The five-year projection seen in

Exhibit 4.8 shows that not only does the system pay for itself, but it continues to provide additional payoff in years 4 and 5 (and presumably ongoing in subsequent years).

EXHIBIT 4.8 **ROI Calculations Worksheet** 0010100100001000011100

	INITIAL	YR. 1	YR. 2	YR. 3	YR. 4	YR. 5	TOTAL
Benefits		$15,000	$35,000	$47,000	$47,000	$47,000	$191,000
Costs	$115,000	$3,200	$4,500	$4,500	$4,500	$4,500	$136,200
Cash Flow	($115,000)	$11,800	$30,500	$42,500	$42,500	$42,500	$54,800
Pay Back		($103,200)	($72,500)	($30,000)	$12,500	$55,000	

Reprinted with permission, Margret\A Consulting, LLC

Cash Flow

Once you have entered all the benefits and costs, you can start to do your ROI calculations. The first calculation may be cash flow. In this case, you assume that the initial costs have been drawn from a capital budget that does not affect the operations budget. However, the ongoing costs will be drawn from the operations budget. Therefore, cash flow is simply the difference between benefits and costs in each year. In the example in Exhibit 4.8, all years had a positive cash flow.

Payback Period

Some providers want to replace their capital reserves, so they are interested in knowing how long it will take to do that. This is the payback period. It is calculated by taking the initial capital expenditure ($115,000 in the example) and continuously subtracting the cash flow for each year. Hence, in year 1, $115,000 minus $11,800 leaves $103,200 to be repaid. Exhibit 4.8 illustrates that it is not until within year 4 that the full amount of the capital has been restored. In other words, the payback period is four years.

The evaluation of the payback period is up to the individual practice. Most EHRs take at least two years to pay back the capital investment, and many can take five or more years. In general, the larger the practice, the more savings are likely and hence the payback is faster. The figures for cost and benefits in Exhibit 4.8 are probably realistic for a three-provider practice.

Internal Rate of Return

Another ROI measure often calculated is the internal rate of return (IRR). This is the rate the investment would earn if you were to put the money into some sort of investment portfolio, such as stocks and bonds. Obviously, the higher the IRR, the more attractive the investment.

For the sample practice shown in Exhibit 4.8, the IRR is 12 percent. Calculating an IRR requires either a financial calculator or use of the IRR function in a spreadsheet. In this case, 12 percent is not bad, considering the way the stock market has been going.

Vendor ROI Calculations

As previously noted, but worth pointing out again, many EHR vendors will run ROI calculations for you. These numbers generally will look better than your own because they often include cost savings from staff reductions that are not real. However, it is important to use vendor cost estimates, and many times vendors have good ideas for where to realize benefits.

▶ Benefits Realization

Most providers will calculate ROI to get some sense of feasibility for the investment. This is very important. However, most providers will rarely take the time later to determine whether that ROI was actually realized. This may be difficult to do, especially due to the many variables that enter into the picture. For example, maybe you implemented an EHR, but then made a decision to start participating in clinical trials. This decision was not based on the capability of the EHR, but the EHR does facilitate it. Should the revenue from the clinical trials participation be included in the EHR benefits realization calculations?

The most important factor after you develop a projected ROI and then acquire and implement the system is to be cognizant of whether benefits are being achieved. You might conduct a perception survey. You could return to your benefits portfolio and actually test some of the assumptions. Obviously, if everyone is "happy," there is little impetus for doing a formal benefits realization study. Still, whether happy or not, at least an informal benefits realization assessment can help you determine if there are problems in the implementation or adoption that could be fixed for better results. For example, if the intent was process improvement in one area for specific revenue increases, and those revenue increases do not seem to be happening, you might want to check whether process improvement is actually being performed. If not, corrective action should be taken. If process improvement is in fact being adopted, then either your original assumptions were incorrect or there are other factors impeding the results from occurring.

A final reason for considering performing some type of benefits realization is to help the practice celebrate its success. Making the investment for an EHR is very significant for most practices. There is risk and a lot of money involved. Part of project planning should be incremental milestones of success that can be celebrated. Even something as simple as a pizza party for all the staff or a letter of commendation in staff files can be a huge morale booster.

▶ Conclusion

This chapter has provided worksheets for creating metrics to describe benefits and calculate costs. It is very important, however, to recognize that benefits will not accrue as anticipated if the systems are not adopted by the users in the manner intended. Many groups have great success with their EHR systems, but other implementations have not succeeded as well. In many cases, a less than desirable result can be attributed to lack of readiness, lack of a planned approach based on the group's readiness, lack of involvement by key stakeholders in planning and selection, and lack of enforcing policies about use.

Change is difficult for everyone, and EHRs require considerable change. Being realistic about the degree of change you can effect and how long it will take will help you estimate a realistic ROI. You don't want to anticipate reaching payback in X years, only to find it is several more years away at your group's actual rate of adoption. In many ways, unrealistic ROI analyses have contributed to concerns about the overall value of EHRs. Most experts recommend being conservative when estimating ROI. However, being too conservative does not help to encourage adoption either. The key to estimating ROI is to gain buy-in from all involved, such that the ROI establishes expectations for meeting goals.

NOTES

1. Ury, A, "The Business Case for an Electronic Medical Record System," *Group Practice Journal*, March 2000.

2. Renner, K, "Electronic Medical Records in the Outpatient Setting," *Medical Group Management Journal*, May/June 1996, 43: 52, 54, 56-57, 74.

3. Dassenko, D and T Slowinski, "Using the CPR to Benefit a Business Office," *Healthcare Financial Management*, July 1995, 49: 68-70, 72-73.

4. Case, J, M Mowry, and E Welebob, "The Nursing Shortage: Can Technology Help?" California HealthCare Foundation, First Consulting Group, June 2002.

5. Bingham, A, "Computerized Patient Records Benefit Physician Offices," *Healthcare Financial Management*, September 1997, 51: 68-70.

6. Stammer, L, "Chart Pulling Brought to Its Knees," *Healthcare Informatics* [serial online], February 2001, 18: 107-108.

7. Mildon, J, and T Cohen, "Drivers in the Electronic Medical Records Market." *Health Management Technology*, May 2001, 22: 14-6, 18.

8. MedicaLogic, "Ambulatory EMR: Establishing a Business Case." Available at www.medicalogic.com/download/www/emr/whitepapers/business_case.pdf.

9. Mildon, J and T. Cohen, op cit.

10. Brandner, B, "EMR ROI and Implementation: Best Practices," *Advance for Health Information Executives*, July 2002, 30-35.

FIVE

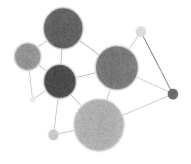

Determining and Managing Your Requirements

The previous chapters helped you to identify your overall objectives and potential return on investment (ROI) from implementing an EHR. This chapter focuses on the detailed specifications you should look for in an EHR product. Your requirements should reflect your vision for the EHR, which in turn drives the types of benefits you projected in your ROI calculations. Hence, defining your requirements is a matter of getting more specific.

THIS CHAPTER ASSISTS you, in particular, in documenting your group's EHR requirements so they may be used for EHR selection criteria and implementation planning. The chapter helps you:

► Understand the relationships among the EHR, practice management (PMS) and/or billing systems, diagnostic systems (e.g., laboratory), other information system applications, and information that can be derived from medical devices;

► Identify your options for an integrated solution vs. independent solutions from multiple vendors;

► Study and describe the features and functions an EHR must have to support your projected benefits;

► Learn how the EHR may require work flow redesign, process improvements, and potentially room layouts and furnishing changes in your practice to achieve your projected benefits; and

▶ Determine if there are special considerations that need to be addressed from your specialty, hospital/practice relationships, and communications with other providers/patients, or to comply with accreditation, licensure, or other legal and regulatory requirements.

▶ System Relationships

An EHR may be a natural progression for your practice from its current PMS, it may be your practice's first major foray into electronic systems, or the acquisition may be intended to integrate multiple disparate systems you already have. Whatever the configuration of your present information systems (IS) environment, it is a good idea to understand the relationships among any existing systems, and your data needs to better prepare you to determine your options for integrating data from multiple sources – for easy access and retrieval of information as well as to provide data for clinical decision support (CDS).

Data Sources and Data Uses

The first step in understanding your present information system(s) relationships and data needs is to make a list of your present data sources and uses. Use the worksheet in Exhibit 5.1 to compile this information. Examples of what might be included are shown in italics. Even if today your practice deals with information only on paper or fax, list all exchanges of data and then explore whether they could be conducted in electronic form.

In using this Sources and Uses of Data Worksheet, be sure to:

▶ List all sources and uses of data.

▷ Sources of data refer to data you capture and record as well as receive from others. These may include data captured in making an appointment for a patient, compiling a patient's medical history, or receiving information about a patient's current medications from a pharmacy. They also include data that may be generated by medical devices you use in the practice, such as ultrasound devices or telemetry devices.

▷ Uses of data refer to the purposes to which you put data – whether for internal documentation, patient care or operational purposes, or for external claims or reporting purposes. Uses of

EXHIBIT 5.1 Sources and Uses of Data Worksheet

SOURCES OF DATA

TYPE	SOURCE(S)	CURRENT MEANS TO CAPTURE OR RETRIEVE DATA						VENDOR APPLICATION				
		PAPER	VERBAL	FAX	WEB	FTP	TRX	NAME	PRODUCT	VERSION	DATE LAST UPGRADE	CURRENT? (Y/N)
Patient appointment	Patient call or visit		X					ABC Co.	QApp	2.3	2002	Y
Medication history	Patient visit	X										
	Pharmacy		X									
Lab results	Community Hospital				X (print out)							
	County Hospital			X								
	XZ Lab					X (print out)						
EOBs	Payers (via clearinghouse)	X										
Refill requests	Retail pharmacies		X									

USES OF DATA

TYPE	USE(S)	CURRENT MEANS TO SUPPLY OR SEND DATA						VENDOR APPLICATION				
		PAPER	VERBAL	FAX	WEB	FTP	TRX	NAME	PRODUCT	VERSION	DATE LAST UPGRADE	CURRENT? (Y/N)
Immunizations	School				X							
	Camp/Sports	X										
	Visa	X										
	Employer					X						
Referral letter	Provider	X										
Claim	Payer						X12 837	ABC Co.	QBill	2.4	2003	Y

data may include referencing lab results to determine the proper dose of a medication, checking an X-ray to determine the exact location of an anomaly, supplying data to payers, sending data to other providers to whom you are referring a patient, or transmitting a report of a communicable disease to the public health department. Remember that data may be used when you talk on the telephone with someone, such as to supply an approval to the pharmacy for a refill or to notify the hospital of an admission. In addition, consider reports you are required to submit with either patient-specific data or aggregate data, such as to state data-reporting agencies, for accreditation and/or credentialing, to cancer or other registries, or for any other purposes. Do you use a coding auditor – if so, how does the auditor access your data? Do you participate in clinical trials or compile data for other research or quality purposes? What other uses of data do you make?

▶ Identify the current means you use to capture or retrieve the data for each source and the means you use to supply or send data for each use. Much will be on paper or via telephone and fax. In some cases, however, you can visit a Web site to retrieve eligibility information or lab results from a hospital. Your office can download data by using a file transfer protocol (FTP). Or, you can send transactions (shown as Trx in Exhibit 5.1) such as claims to a payer or receive transactions such as a batch of explanations of benefits (EOBs) from a payer.

▶ Make sure your lists of sources and uses of data include data that relate to your practice, even if not necessarily related to a specific patient. For example, your practice management system (PMS) may have the following applications: billing, patient appointment and registration, and accounting. You may have a separate time and attendance system, dictation system, and e-prescribing system. You may also have various word processing, spreadsheet, and e-mail applications.

▶ Include any knowledge sources to which you subscribe. For example, you can download formulary information from a payer or pharmacy benefits manager (PBM), subscribe to a drug knowledge database service, periodically retrieve clinical guidelines from the Agency for Healthcare Research and Quality (AHRQ), American College of Physicians (ACP), Physicians' Information and Education Resource (PIER), or other sources. Or, you can routinely check a

Web site for the International Classification of Diseases, Ninth Revision, Clinical Modification (ICD-9-CM), or Current Procedural Terminology® (CPT®) coding assistance.

As you list your sources and uses of data, be as specific as you can. This list will ultimately serve as your checklist to make sure that your EHR can accommodate all the data you want to capture or use. It will help ensure that the product you select can help you receive data from applicable sources or send data to appropriate users. During system implementation and testing, you will also want to make sure that the data can actually be sent and/or received as you intend.

Format and Transmission of Data

Once you have listed all the sources and uses of data, you may also find it helpful to describe the various formats of the data that come to you or that you submit. For example, instead of merely indicating that you send claims via transactions, you may find it helpful to indicate the standard protocol you use, such as Accredited Standards Committee (ASC) X12N 837.

The Health Insurance Portability and Accountability Act of 1996 (HIPAA) requires use of the X12N 837 standard if you are sending claims electronically (either directly or via a clearinghouse), but there are additional X12N standards under HIPAA, as well as other standards for other types of data, that you may be using. For example, if you use e-prescribing, does your e-prescribing device transmit a fax to the pharmacy or does it send a transaction using the National Council for Prescription Drug Programs (NCPDP) SCRIPT standard? If you are able to retrieve X-ray images from a hospital, does the transmission of the image follow the Digital Imaging and Communications in Medicine (DICOM) standard protocol? If so, then the image is a digital image, and it can be integrated into other digital data in your systems. If the image transmission is not DICOM, then the image it is merely a picture – you will still be able to see it, but you won't be able to process it as you would a digital image.

You may not have the immediate answers to these questions, but you may want to investigate such issues because vendor products that comply with standard protocols help ensure that systems can exchange data. For example, you may have a patient scheduling system from one vendor and a patient billing system from another vendor. If they are both Health Level Seven® (HL7®) compliant, an interface can probably be written that would allow demographic data from the scheduling system to be passed to the billing system. However, if either of the systems are not HL7 compliant, writing an interface for such exchange of data between the systems will be much more difficult, if not impossible. When systems use standard protocols and have interfaces written for exchange of data, the systems are said to be "interoperable."

Exhibit 5.2 lists the interoperability standards most commonly used in EHR and other health information technology (HIT) systems for provider offices.

EXHIBIT 5.2 Commonly Used Standards and Their Purposes

STANDARD	PURPOSE
ASC X12:	
▶ 837	▶ Claim
▶ 835	▶ Remittance advice (e.g., explanation of benefits, or EOB)
▶ 270/271	▶ Eligibility inquiry and response
▶ 276/277	▶ Claim status inquiry and response
▶ 278	▶ Prior authorization
▶ 277/275	▶ Claims attachment*
▶ 834	▶ Health plan enrollment/disenrollment**
▶ 820	▶ Health plan premium payment**
ASTM International Continuity of Care Record (CCR)	Standard protocol for exchange of content for patient referrals
DICOM	Standard protocol for exchange of health care images, such as X-rays
HL7	Standard protocols for exchange of data among health care IS components, such as a PMS and an EHR system, or between a laboratory information system and computerized provider order entry system
NCPDP:	
▶ Telecommunication Standard	▶ Retail pharmacy claims, eligibility, and remittance advice
▶ SCRIPT Standard	▶ Prescriptions from providers to retail pharmacies

* This standard was required by the HIPAA legislation and is available for voluntary usage, although a specific regulation was not promulgated at the time this book was published.
** These are HIPAA transactions available for your use as an employer.

Reprinted with permission, Margret\A Consulting, LLC

Data Flow Analysis

Another reason for compiling a list of data sources and uses is to help you determine how information technology (IT) can help you capture and process the information better. For this, you may want to extend the Data Sources and Uses Worksheet by the additional columns shown in Exhibit 5.3 on the next page. (This can easily be accomplished by setting up a spreadsheet using the column headings shown in Exhibits 5.1 and 5.3. Some cells have been filled in with examples in italics.)

In using this Analysis of Data Flow Worksheet, be sure to:

▶ *Record information about any current electronic format.* If a standard is used, identify it. If data are received or sent electronically, but via proprietary means, indicate "proprietary" on the spreadsheet. It is a good idea to indicate if you are sending or receiving data in batch or real-time mode. Batch refers to collecting data or transactions and sending or receiving them all at one time, such as daily, weekly, or monthly. Real time refers to the fact that you can receive data at the same time as you make a request for the data. Also indicate whether there is a fee associated with sending or receiving a transmission of data.

▶ *Determine and record future plans.* Indicate what data you want to accommodate in your EHR or other HIT and the timeline. If you determine that data cannot be supplied to you electronically now, but can at some time in the future, indicate the amount of time you may need to wait. Also indicate the standard you expect to use (which may be the same as that you are currently using). Record any special comments that will help you in your planning. Finally, rank the importance (high, medium, low) of each of your plans.

If you are currently receiving or recording the data via paper, telephone, or fax, analyze whether it is feasible to receive the data electronically. In the example shown in Exhibit 5.3, patient appointments are made via an appointment system. The provider will want to make sure it integrates with the EHR being acquired. This will probably be a high-priority requirement. Also in the example, the patient's medication history captured during a visit is currently recorded on paper, so it will probably be a high priority to have the capability to record medication history in the EHR being acquired.

If you are currently retrieving data via Web access or FTP, analyze whether it is feasible to receive the data in an electronic transaction that can be received more directly by your information system.

EXHIBIT 5.3 Analysis of Data Flow Worksheet

SOURCES OF DATA		ELECTRONIC FORMAT				FUTURE PLANS				
TYPE	SOURCE(S)	STANDARD	BATCH	REAL-TIME	FEE?	INFORMATION TECHNOLOGY	TIME LINE	MEANS	COMMENTS	REQUIRED? & PRIORITY (H-M-L)
Patient appointment	Patient call or visit					Integrate with EHR	Now	HL7	ABC Co. is HL7 compliant	H
Medication history	Patient visit					Include in EHR	Now	HL7	"	H
	Pharmacy					PBM Trx	2 Yrs.	?	Requires fee	L
Lab results	Community Hospital									
	County Hospital					None			Will need to scan	H
	XZ Lab	X								
EOBs	Payers (via clearinghouse)									
Refill requests	Retail pharmacies		X			Electronic prescribing				

USES OF DATA		ELECTRONIC FORMAT				FUTURE PLANS				
TYPE	USE(S)	STANDARD	BATCH	REAL-TIME	FEE?	INFORMATION TECHNOLOGY	TIME LINE	MEANS	COMMENTS	REQUIRED? & PRIORITY (H-M-L)
Immunizations	School									
	Camp/Sports									
	Visa									
	Employer									
Referral letters	Provider					Integrate EHR with CCR	Now	ASTM		M
Claims	Payer	X12N 837	Nightly		$0.25/Trx					

Reprinted with permission, Marget\A Consulting, LLC

Consider all possible sources of data. For example, instead of waiting for the pharmacy to call you that there may be a contraindication with another medication, you may want to subscribe to a medication history service offered by a PBM, which, for a transaction fee, can provide a daily download of current medication history for each patient. Even if you find this interesting and potentially valuable, you may decide it is lower (L) on your list of priorities for the EHR.

If the source of the data is external to you and does not currently have the capability to supply data electronically, make a note concerning the source's plans for the future. In the example, the county hospital is able to send you only a fax of lab results. Inquire if it has plans to open a Web portal, such as the community hospital has. The county hospital may not, but at least you will know that you will still need to be able to retrieve documents via fax and potentially can scan them into your system.

Similarly, indicate how you would like to supply or send data to others. For example, if you are currently sending referral letters to other providers, you may want to indicate that you would like the EHR you acquire to have the capability to supply data to a CCR by using the ASTM International standard data content. Once again, rate the priority for this feature. In the example, this was rated medium (M).

▶ Integrated vs. Independent Solutions

With the EHR ideally permitting capture of data from multiple sources, different "source systems" need to be able to contribute data to the EHR. How that happens is an important consideration in what you are buying as an EHR – and part of the reason to analyze your current data sources and uses, as described above.

In simplest terms, an EHR that captures data from multiple sources does so in one of two basic ways:

1. All data flows into a repository. The repository allows direct access to all data and can also make data from different sources available for processing into meaningful information. What you are buying as an information system, then, is a repository – which is software that manages a sophisticated database, software that facilitates data entry and viewing, and software to further process the data in the repository.

2. Multiple source systems are either fully integrated or interfaced to make it appear to the user that the data are coming from a single system. In this model, the "EHR system" helps the user capture and retrieve data. When the user wants access to data, the EHR system retrieves it from the respective source system or systems, processes the data, and provides views of it to the user.

The two models may appear to produce the same end results – the user gets the needed data – but there actually are very big differences between integrated systems and interfaced systems, as well as between the integrated/interfaced model and the repository model.

Repository Model

The repository model is generally ideal for use when a practice has multiple, disparate information systems, or expects to receive data from multiple disparate sources. In addition to being a central place to house this data, a repository is a powerful source to tap for processing data in many different ways. Exhibit 5.4 provides one example of how effective a repository model EHR can be when there are multiple source systems.

In Exhibit 5.4, the patient appointment is made in a scheduling system that transmits demographic data to the repository. The provider subscribes to a medication history service, available from a consortium of PBMs, which sends a download every night to the provider's repository based on the patient schedule for the next day. The provider also has available from this service formulary information from the patients' payers. Lab data has already been transmitted to the provider's repository as it became available. When the patient is seen, then, the provider uses the EHR to capture a complete history and physical, makes a diagnosis, and is aided in selecting potential drugs from the latest drug information available through a drug knowledge base (DKB) to which the provider subscribes. All data in the repository are processed to consider the patient's medication history, lab values, indications, payer rules, and efficacy (Eff) of the drug from various clinical trials. In the example shown in Exhibit 5.4, the provider is able to review five potential drugs in the class selected. Drug 2 requires a prior authorization (P.A.) from the payer. The provider can choose to electronically transmit a request for prior authorization, but perhaps decides, based on cost and efficacy, that two other drugs, 3 and 5, are just as good candidates for the patient. (Drugs 1 and 4 have been eliminated due to a potential contraindication and allergen, respectively.) Information on relative cost and efficacy for drugs 3 and 5 is reviewed, making the choice clear that

EXHIBIT 5.4   Repository Model Example   1001010010000010001100

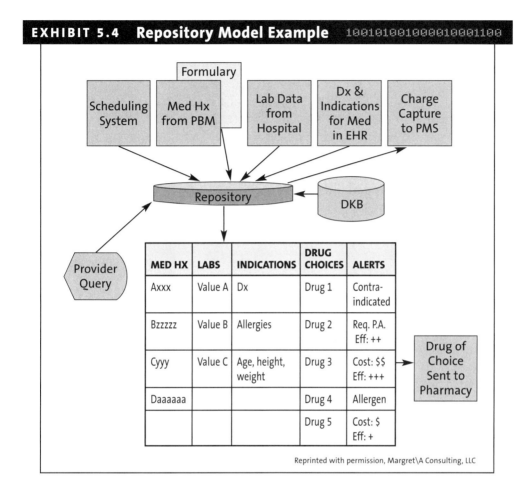

Reprinted with permission, Margret\A Consulting, LLC

despite the somewhat greater cost, the efficacy of drug 3 is far better than drug 5.

The repository model is commonly the model of choice for large provider groups and hospitals, but it does require knowledgeable IT staff to manage it. For smaller provider practices, the repository model is generally a more sophisticated form of EHR.

Integrated Model

The integrated model is generally offered by a single vendor. Rather than separate source systems, the vendor has built components that have all been developed using the same technical platform and are designed to work together. Many PMSs and EHR systems for provider practices have been designed in this way.

The integrated model uses a database structure that manages the data as it is captured and used within the various components. The most important advantage to an integrated solution is the simplicity of its architecture while still providing solid functionality. A disadvantage of an integrated system is that if the practice needs special functionality that the vendor does not support, it can be difficult to interface another system with the fully integrated one. This is often because the tight integration is accomplished through proprietary protocols.

Exhibit 5.5 illustrates an integrated model in which the PMS and EHR functions are fully integrated, but the e-prescribing function is separate. In this case, much – but not all – of the information or information processing capability exists. The provider obtains the medication history exclusively from the patient – who may have forgotten about taking one of the medications. The provider has access to the latest information on drug choices, efficacy, and relative cost from the e-prescribing system, but must integrate that knowledge with the information captured during the encounter. As can be seen in this example, by not knowing about a drug the patient is taking and therefore not having it available in the same system for an alert to a contraindication, the provider may choose a drug that actually is wrong for the patient. The pharmacy – which often has medication history from payers in its system – will probably catch this oversight and call the provider, but, obviously, the chance exists that the pharmacy does not have the information either, which can result in a medication error and potential for an adverse drug event.

Interfaced Model

The interfaced model is one in which different systems can exchange data through specifically written software, called interfaces. This can work well enough if the different systems were designed in compliance with standard protocols. In general, however, the interfaced model does not afford as robust a processing capability as either the integrated model or the repository model.

If systems are designed without standard protocols, or protocols are only loosely followed, the data do not pass as smoothly as possible through the systems and perhaps cannot be processed together as easily, if at all. As previously noted, many PMSs and even some EHR systems for provider practices have been developed without using standard protocols. Note also that just because one vendor offers both a PMS and an EHR, the systems are not

EXHIBIT 5.5   Integrated Model Example   1001010010000100001100

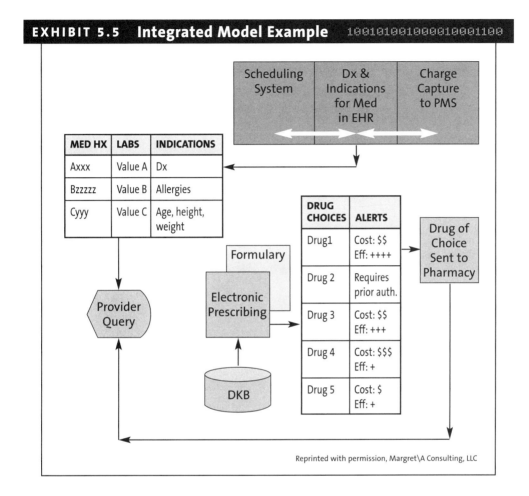

Reprinted with permission, Margret\A Consulting, LLC

necessarily integrated. If the vendor developed one of the systems and acquired another company to complement the product offerings, it is possible that the two systems can only be interfaced.

Exhibit 5.6 on the next page illustrates the interfaced model, once again using the example of selecting a drug for a patient.

In the example in Exhibit 5.6, notice that a new drug not identified in either of the other two models is introduced. Perhaps the person capturing the drug information misidentified the patient because the PMS is not integrated with the EHR. Although the result is the same as the integrated model, it could have been different.

EXHIBIT 5.6 Interfaced Model Example

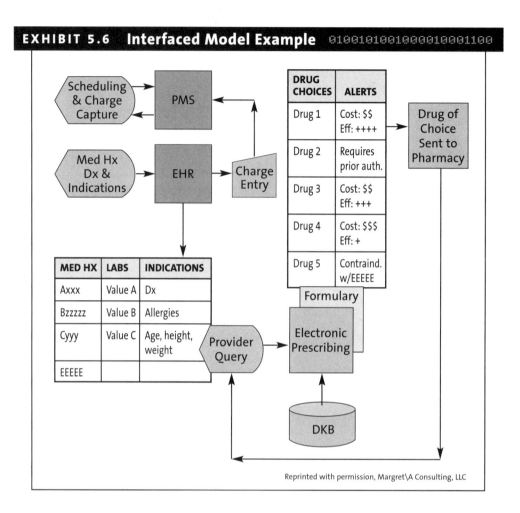

Reprinted with permission, Margret\A Consulting, LLC

Solution Decision

Bear in mind that errors can occur in any of the three models. Just because the illustrations demonstrate that errors are more likely to occur in the integrated and interfaced models does not necessarily mean that they will, or that the same types of errors illustrated will occur. The exhibits are intended only to illustrate that the risk is potentially greater as you move from a repository structure to an interfaced one.

Your decision about the model you acquire depends on many factors. In part, your existing systems may contribute to your decision making. Your future plans must also be considered. If you are satisfied with one or more information systems that you have now and they are HL7 compliant, you can consider the repository or interface model. Your choice then depends primarily on your future plans. Do you anticipate expanding into other specialty services that may require the special features and functions of a separate system? For example, someone with an internal medicine practice today may have little need for integrating X-ray images through a picture archiving and communication system (PACS). But what if that provider decides to expand into general surgery or add a cardiology subspecialty? In such situations, the repository option offers the best way to add disparate systems. Alternatively, if that provider's long-term plans call for only more of the same, an existing or a new vendor may offer an EHR that can be interfaced with the other systems very well.

If your present systems are not HL7 compliant and your vendor does not offer an EHR component that is integrated, then your choices generally are between a repository model and replacement of current systems along with an EHR.

In considering the repository structure, be sure you thoroughly evaluate the ability of the systems to contribute data to the repository. A repository requires structured data using, at a minimum, a common data dictionary, and ideally a standard vocabulary.

Structured data refers to data that are captured as discrete data elements, rather than in a narrative stream of words. Unstructured data are simply narrative or text-based data not related to a data dictionary or standard vocabulary. Exhibit 5.7 on the next page illustrates the difference between structured and unstructured data.

Using structured data with a standard vocabulary is the key to a successful EHR. For example, referring to the drug selection example from the previous exhibits, if you currently subscribe to a drug knowledge database from vendor X, but the EHR you are considering comes with a drug knowledge database from vendor Y, you could be faced with two different ways of naming drugs. Most drug knowledge databases are based on the Food and Drug Administration (FDA) National Drug Code (NDC) system. However, NDCs are primarily used to describe packaged drugs a pharmacy would retain in its inventory. Most clinicians prefer to prescribe drugs using a clinical drug vocabulary rather than a packaged drug vocabulary. Drug knowledge database vendors help make that translation occur. If, however, the drug knowledge database vendor does not use a standard clinical drug vocabulary (such as RxNorm, which is being developed for this purpose), confusion could result.

EXHIBIT 5.7 **Structured vs. Unstructured Data** 0010000100001100

STRUCTURED DATA	UNSTRUCTURED DATA
Social History: ▶ Alcohol ___ Ounces per day ▶ Tobacco ___ Cigarettes per day or equivalent	*Social History:* *The patient does not smoke, but has three beers a day.*
This example collects precise information in discrete form.	This example collects imprecise information in a stream of narrative text.
A computer can be programmed to process this data to compare, for example, smokers against non-smokers, persons who consume 4 ounces of alcohol a day against those who consume 12 ounces per day, etc.	It is difficult for most computer systems to be able to process this data. For example, when the computer separates each word in the sentence, the word "smoke" could refer to a patient who smokes cigarettes or to a patient who has been exposed to smoke from a fire.

Reprinted with permission, Margret\A Consulting, LLC

Similarly, if the EHR vendor uses a proprietary vocabulary for identifying the values for data to be collected in a structured history and physical examination, the data captured may not be comparable with data from another system that uses a different proprietary vocabulary, or even a standard vocabulary, such as SNOMED CT® (see Chapter 2, EHR Technology).

Much like the standard protocols for interoperability, the functioning of a repository depends on standard vocabularies for data comparability. If data are not comparable, you may not be able to process the data against rules to supply alerts and reminders and other clinical decision support. In the drug selection example, the computer would not be able to compare the list of drugs you capture as the medication history against a payer's formulary or efficacy information from a drug knowledge database if each of the sets of drugs used a different vocabulary. (This is much like translating information from one language to another. Sometimes meaning gets lost in the translation in going from, for example, French to German or Arabic to Chinese.)

A note of caution should be made, however, concerning structured data. The primary advantage of structured data is for the data to be processed by the computer. However, there is a balance between the extensive time required to check off such precise data and the value returned. Furthermore, some unusual cases may exist that only narrative data can describe. Structured data may not always make the data as "rich" in meaning as narrative data. For example, in Exhibit 5.7, the amount of alcohol consumed is not very precise in the narrative form, but the physician is able to record the type of alcohol (beer) consumed. This may be useful information to the physician for subsequent visits – perhaps inquiring of the patient if beer continues to be consumed. Many EHR products attempt to combine the best of both structured and narrative data, so that perhaps the actual amount of alcohol consumed can be captured, but the type of alcohol could be recorded in a narrative field when desired.

▶ Features and Functions

Your decision about the architecture of the EHR has a bearing on the features and functions the EHR can support. In general, the repository model can support the most functions and the interface model has the potential for supporting the least. As previously noted, however, what can actually be supported is highly variable. A full integrated model may work well, but have fewer of the features and functions that you want.

Resources to Identify Functions

Various resources can assist you in identifying the specific functionality you want. Your primary resource, of course, should be your own list of sources and uses of data, but other resources can be helpful because they can give you ideas for how you can improve current information handling.

Many potential users of EHRs in a practice may not be aware of the full range of functions an EHR can provide. However, looking at lists of functions can also be like the proverbial "kid in the candy store." You may find you want everything, whether or not you truly will use the functions. Once again, your own list of sources and uses of data should enable you to evaluate what functions are truly important.

Exhibit 5.8 on the next page lists some of the resources available to help you identify functions and what to expect from them.

Target Functions

To help you organize your own set of functional requirements that are most important for you, Exhibit 5.9 shown on pages 132–34 provides a worksheet

EXHIBIT 5.8   Feature/Function Resources   0010100100000010001100

RESOURCES	DESCRIPTION
Institute of Medicine (IOM): ▶ *Computer-based Patient Records: An Essential Technology for Health Care*, National Academy Press, 1991, 1997 ▶ Key Capabilities of an Electronic Health Record System, July 31, 2003.	▶ An early report on what has now come to be identified as EHR; provides justification for and fundamental description of EHR. ▶ Up-to-date list of features and functions characterized by general care settings; focuses on care delivery functions; does not address infra-structure functions.
Health Level Seven (HL7): ▶ EHR Functional Descriptors, Draft Standard for Trial Use (DSTU), July 27, 2004	▶ Visionary description of all potential functions for an EHR, irrespective of care setting; may be the basis for EHR product certification.
Trade publications' annual directories of EHR vendors	Quick means to identify vendors and make rudimentary comparisons on preselected characteristics, based on self-reported data.
Vendor Web sites	Marketing material designed to describe products' best features; demos may be available that can be used for initial education about how EHRs work.
Trade shows	Also marketing opportunity to set forth products' best features; sales personnel may not be able to provide in-depth responses to questions, but this is a good way to see demos.
Specialty society recommendations	Depending on society policy, may provide a "consumer reports" perspective; helps identify products that meet unique needs of certain specialties.

Reprinted with permission, Margret\A Consulting, LLC

on which you can identify functions that match your requirements (as identified from the Analysis of Data Flow Worksheet in Exhibit 5.3). This worksheet combines functions identified in the Institute of Medicine (IOM) patient safety reports, HL7's Draft Standard for Trial Use (DSTU), and various other sources as they most closely match provider practice needs. The worksheet can be modified to fit any other source of functionality you choose to reference.

Once you have settled on your own functional list, it can then be used as part of your requirements specification in your request for proposal (RFP) as you approach vendors, and as a checklist in evaluating how likely each vendor product you review may be able to contribute to your defined benefits expectations.

▶ Translating Functionality into Benefits

"Buy this EHR and You Won't Have to Change Your Processes."

This message has been in various EHR vendor advertisements in one form or another. It sounds attractive – you'll get all the benefits of an EHR without making any changes. Unfortunately, spending significant resources to make no process improvements is an unwise investment.

It should be obvious that the functions you seek in an EHR will contribute to achieving your objectives only if current work flows and processes are evaluated and necessary changes are made. Yet it is these changes that are the most difficult to accomplish. In fact, even some of the most well-intentioned will attempt to customize the new EHR so that it reflects current processes – which are not producing your intended benefits.

Preparing your practice for change and managing this change are critical steps in making the functions of the EHR work for you. The EHR can – and should – change the way you do things to produce your desired benefits.

Although you don't want to introduce change for change's sake or where the outcome is not desirable, you need to give the EHR product you acquire a chance. You need to study and learn how the system will impact your work flow and processes, work with users to make the changes, and assess the results. An old adage that is much more apropos to the EHR is: "You pay for what you get." The "pay" here is both in actual out-of-pocket expenses for the EHR system and the time you invest in making the right selection, fitting it into your practice, and fitting your work and processes into it.

Work Flow Redesign

Work flow refers to the sequence of steps taken to accomplish a process. Typically, work flow refers to passing work from one person to the next,

EXHIBIT 5.9 Functional Requirements 101001010010000010001100

COMMON FUNCTIONAL REQUIREMENTS	PRIORITY (FROM ANALYSIS OF DATA FLOW WORKSHEET)	EXPECTED BENEFIT	VENDOR ASSESSMENT (RATE ON SCALE OF 1 TO 5: 1 = DOES NOT PROVIDE FUNCTIONALITY TO 5 = PROVIDES BEST FUNCTIONALITY)				
			A	B	C	D	E
Identify and locate a patient							
Manage patient demographics							
Identify patient relationships							
Manage problem list							
Manage medication list							
Manage allergy and adverse reaction list							
Capture patient history							
Manage diagnostic studies results							
Summarize health record							
Manage clinical documentation and notes							
Capture key health data							
Capture external clinical documents							
Capture patient-originated data							
Manage patient-specific care plans, guidelines, and protocols							
Capture variances from standard care plans, guidelines, and protocols							
Provide patient-specific instructions							
Manage medication formularies							
Write prescriptions							
Drug, food, allergy interaction checking							
Patient-specific dosing and warnings							
Order diagnostic tests							
Order referrals							
Manage consents and authorizations							

EXHIBIT 5.9 Functional Requirements *continued* 001000010001100

COMMON FUNCTIONAL REQUIREMENTS	PRIORITY (FROM ANALYSIS OF DATA FLOW WORKSHEET)	EXPECTED BENEFIT	VENDOR ASSESSMENT (RATE ON SCALE OF 1 TO 5: 1 = DOES NOT PROVIDE FUNCTIONALITY TO 5 = PROVIDES BEST FUNCTIONALITY)				
			A	B	C	D	E
Manage patient advance directives							
Receive support from standard assessments							
Receive support from patient context-enabled assessments							
Receive information on most cost-effective services, referrals, devices, etc. to recommend to patient							
Support service requests and claims processing							
Support management of patient groups or populations							
Support research protocols							
Support for health maintenance, preventive care, and wellness							
Support for notification and response from external sources							
Access clinical guidance							
Schedule and manage clinical tasks							
Support secure electronic communication							
Support communication and presentation of data captured from medical devices							
Enable transfer of data to notifiable registries							
Provide a current directory of provider information							
Manage provider identifiers							
Enable de-identification of protected health information when necessary							
Enable printout of information when necessary							

continued next page

EXHIBIT 5.9 **Functional Requirements** *continued* 0010000100001100

COMMON FUNCTIONAL REQUIREMENTS	PRIORITY (FROM ANALYSIS OF DATA FLOW WORKSHEET)	EXPECTED BENEFIT	VENDOR ASSESSMENT (RATE ON SCALE OF 1 TO 5: 1 = DOES NOT PROVIDE FUNCTIONALITY TO 5 = PROVIDES BEST FUNCTIONALITY)				
			A	B	C	D	E
Support measurement and monitoring of care for relevant purposes							
Automatically generate administrative and financial data from clinical record							
Provide rules-driven financial and administrative coding assistance							
Enable specialized views of data							
Support remote access and health care services							
Manage patient reminders							
Provide secure authentication							
Provide access management and audit trail services							
Enforce patient privacy and confidentiality							
Ensure integrity, data retention, and availability							
Maintain versioning of health informatics and terminology standards							
Support interoperability through compliance with interchange standards and agreements							
Manage work flows, including work queues, personnel, rooms, and equipment							
Other:							
Other:							

Reference Sources: HL7 EHR System Functional Model DSTU, 2004; and Institute of Medicine of the National Academies (IOM) "Data Standards for Patient Safety" project reports.

Reprinted with permission, Margret\A Consulting, LLC

such as from the receptionist to the nurse, from the nurse to physician, from the physician to the biller, and so forth. An EHR will eliminate, for example, having to move charts from a file room to the registration area when the patient has an appointment scheduled.

A number of classic tools are available to evaluate current work flow and determine how the work flow may need to be changed due to EHR implementation or how the EHR needs to be customized to fit into your work flow.

PHYSICAL LAYOUT

From the physical facility perspective, the most important considerations for implementing an EHR are the location of the workstations and technical infrastructure.

Chapter 2 stresses that workstations – whether they are desktop or handheld devices – need to be ubiquitous for successful use of an EHR. Use a layout of each practice location and identify where each type of device needs to be located. Be sure to include all registration areas, conference rooms, offices, examining rooms, and so forth.

If there is insufficient room for a desktop computer in examining rooms, then consider handheld devices. However, a handheld or wireless device still needs a location in the examining room to be placed while administering to a patient. This temporary location should not put the device at risk for falling or be a place where liquids could spill onto it. You may consider installing a shelf where the device can be placed temporarily.

Consider also how any workstation or other human-computer interface (HCI) device is used in relationship to the patient. Many providers express concern that they don't want the device to "come between" them and the patient. Interestingly, however, many providers are unaware of how frequently they have their backs to their patients as they are documenting in their paper charts. It may be prudent to "role play" the relationship of provider and patient in the exam room to see what works best. Literally draw a picture of the exam room – to scale, such as in Exhibit 5.10 shown on the next page – to determine where devices should be placed.

In the sample layout in Exhibit 5.10, the provider may currently use the desk marked A to make a record in the patient's chart. Note that this puts

EXHIBIT 5.10 Layout Considerations for Workstations 10001100

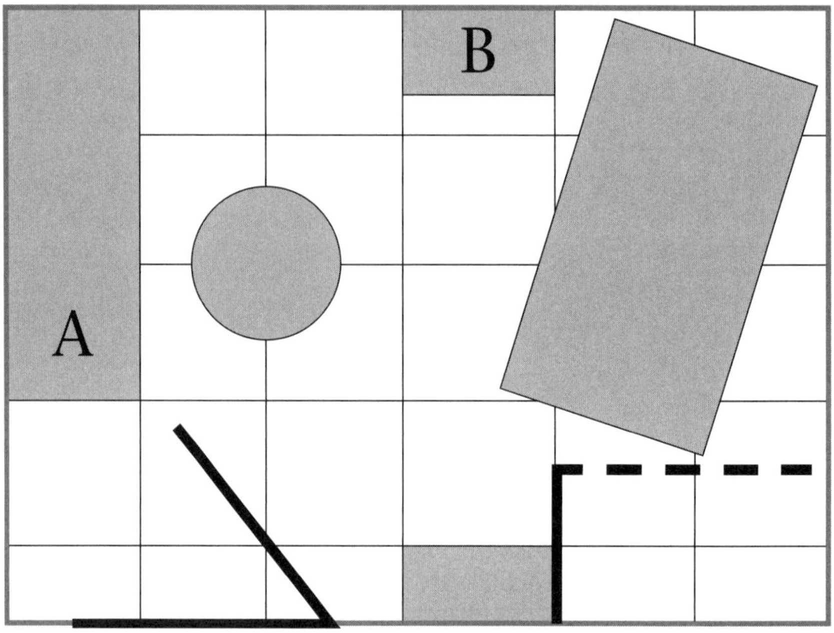

Reprinted with permission, Margret\A Consulting, LLC

the provider's back to the patient during that activity. In determining the location of a workstation to overcome the issue of not facing the patient, however, consider the following:

- ▶ Cabinet B is quite small and very likely also used for instrument placement, so there probably is not enough room for a workstation, or even a temporary location for a portable device;

- ▶ Desk A puts the provider's back to the patient, not unlike current usage, but does afford the patient the view of a workstation screen, which may be desirable;

- ▶ Desk A is quite narrow and may not hold a normal PC workstation, which means that the monitor has to be one of the newer, flat panel types. Even at that, the keyboard and monitor may not fit there;

- ▶ If a portable device were used by the provider, the device could be in any location as the provider sits on the swivel chair, and Desk A could probably serve as a temporary holding area, unless it is typically cluttered with books, telephone, etc.; and

- ▶ Some practices also mount notebook computers or tablets to carts.

As Chapter 2, EHR Technology, notes: Servers, network devices, and cabling need to be accommodated somewhere. In the past, a multi-purpose room may have been used as a lunch room, conference location, and storage area for computer equipment. Due to the mission-critical nature of the EHR, however, it is best to find a separate location for this equipment. For example, some offices use closets or they wall off an area of a larger room. Just be sure that this area has sufficient ventilation and that power is not disrupted by heating and cooling issues, overuse of electrical outlets, and so on. Other heavy power users, such as refrigerators, microwave ovens, or photocopiers, should not be in the same location.

FLOW CHARTS

In addition to the location of devices within the physical space, consider the flow of work within the practice. The introduction to this section notes that in the past, paper charts frequently were passed between one person and the next or from one department to another.

Although the EHR should (at least ultimately) eliminate the need for pulling charts, you should understand how the process of passing off work from one person to another will occur in the EHR environment. For example, when a patient is brought to the examining room, a nurse may log onto the system, enter vital signs and other information, and then will need to log off. The physician will then need to log on again. Some practices find constant logging on and off cumbersome and decide to leave a system logged on at all times under one person's log-in. In addition to this being a violation of HIPAA's Privacy and Security Rules, which make it clear that each user must have a unique user identification and password or other means of authentication, this process also introduces other risks: A continuously logged on system does not afford accountability for people's actions. A risk exists that an unauthorized person may use the open log-in to write a prescription, to gain unauthorized access to information, or even to alter information. Ways to overcome such issues include each caregiver having a unique handheld device or activating log-on via a biometric means.

Many other work flows are positively impacted by the EHR. A good way to evaluate how an EHR may change work flows is to list current steps in a work flow and compare that list to the list of steps that would be used in the EHR. This method not only serves to recognize the differences but to establish expectations for how new work flow must occur to achieve the benefits of an EHR.

Exhibit 5.11 illustrates a step list for a typical prescription refill in a practice with paper charts. The 21 steps not only involve significant unproductive work, such as physically carrying the chart from one place to another, but also represent a multi-hour-long process from the time the telephone call is received until the prescription is ordered by phone or mailed to the patient. Further, this is accomplished without any automated checking of potential allergies or contraindications with other current medications, which would be included in the EHR.

In planning the flow of steps this same procedure would take in an EHR environment, do not replicate the unnecessary steps or plan for new functions or additional technology that may extend beyond the EHR. For example, many practices have taken advantage of the EHR to get a telephone system that routes refill requests directly to a nurse who handles all incoming refill calls directly. The nurse is able to access the patient's record while on the telephone with the pharmacy or patient, and either approve the refill based on the information already documented in the chart or send a note electronically for the physician to review the request and process it, also electronically. Not only does this expedite the refill function, but it enhances patient safety and improves patient satisfaction.

As noted, such a listing illustrates the critical importance of agreement to this work flow and responsibility for responding to electronic messages.

In addition to step lists, a flowchart can be an effective way to illustrate where delays and bottlenecks occur in the present process and show how that may be changed with an EHR. A flowchart can more readily illustrate decision points and flow of information. Exhibit 5.12 on page 141 illustrates the same steps as the current process in Exhibit 5.11, but in flowchart form.

Process Design and Improvement

In addition to work flow redesign, which typically addresses the sequence of tasks between people or departments, process improvement refers to the systematic actions an individual takes to perform a function. For example, process improvement may include how a provider reads a medical record, what information is recorded on a prescription, or the decision making that goes into selecting the appropriate service level code for an encounter.

In selecting an EHR, it is very important to understand the processes supported by the system and to have the ability to make changes in those processes where necessary. The caution still applies, however, to ensure

EXHIBIT 5.11   Example 1 of Prescription Refill Work Flow Step List

CURRENT WORK FLOW	EHR WORK FLOW	E-PRESCRIBING WORK FLOW
1. Patient or pharmacy calls physician practice for a refill.	1. Patient calls physician practice for a refill.	1. Pharmacy transmits refill request to e-prescribing device.
2. Support staff writes down the message (live or from voice mail).	2. Nurse accepts call.	
3. Written message sits in out-basket.		
4. Written message is carried to medical records.		
5. Patient's paper chart pulled, if it is found.		
6. Chart sits in out-box.		
7. Chart is carried to nurse.		
8. Nurse reviews chart containing medications previously ordered by this provider and determines if current test results are present or need to be requested.	3. Nurse reviews chart online, which includes a list of all current medications prescribed by any provider, all current lab results, refill status, and other information to approve refill, or nurse requests physician review of refill request.	
9. Nurse writes recommendation for physician.		
10. Chart with nurse's note sits in out-basket.		
11. Chart is carried to physician's office.		
12. Chart waits for physician's review.		
13. Physician reads note and chart.	4. Physician is alerted to refill requests and reviews nurse's recommendations.	2. Physician is alerted to refill requests.

continued next page

EXHIBIT 5.11 Example 1 of Prescription Refill Work Flow Step List *cont.*

CURRENT WORK FLOW	EHR WORK FLOW	E-PRESCRIBING WORK FLOW
14. Physician evaluates information, writes prescription, or requests appointment or diagnostic test.	5. Physician evaluates information, writes and transmits prescription to pharmacy, or transmits request for appointment or diagnostic test to clerical staff to notify patient.	3. Physician may route to nurse or review chart online, which includes list of all current medications prescribed by any provider, all current lab results, refill status, and other information to approve refill.
15. Physician documents in the chart or dictates for transcription.		
16. Chart and prescription sit in out-basket.		
17. Chart and prescription carried to nurse.		
18. Nurse either (a) puts the prescription in an envelope addressed to patient or (b) calls pharmacy.	6. Nurse or physician transmits prescription refill to pharmacy of patient's choice.	4. Nurse or physician transmits prescription refill to pharmacy of patient's choice.
19. Chart sits in out-box.		
20. Chart is carried to medical records.		
21. Medical records files the chart.		

Reprinted with permission, Boundary Information Group and Margret\A Consulting, LLC

process changes imposed by the EHR are evaluated critically so you don't make changes that return the processes to their "old" ways. The idea is to improve processes through the use of IT.

Some considerations regarding process redesign relative to EHR systems include the following:

▶ *Screen layout.* This refers to how the data to be captured or retrieved are presented. Is the layout of the screen and its various components intuitive? Can a person learn to work with the data on

EXHIBIT 5.12   Example 2 of Prescription Refill Work Flow Chart

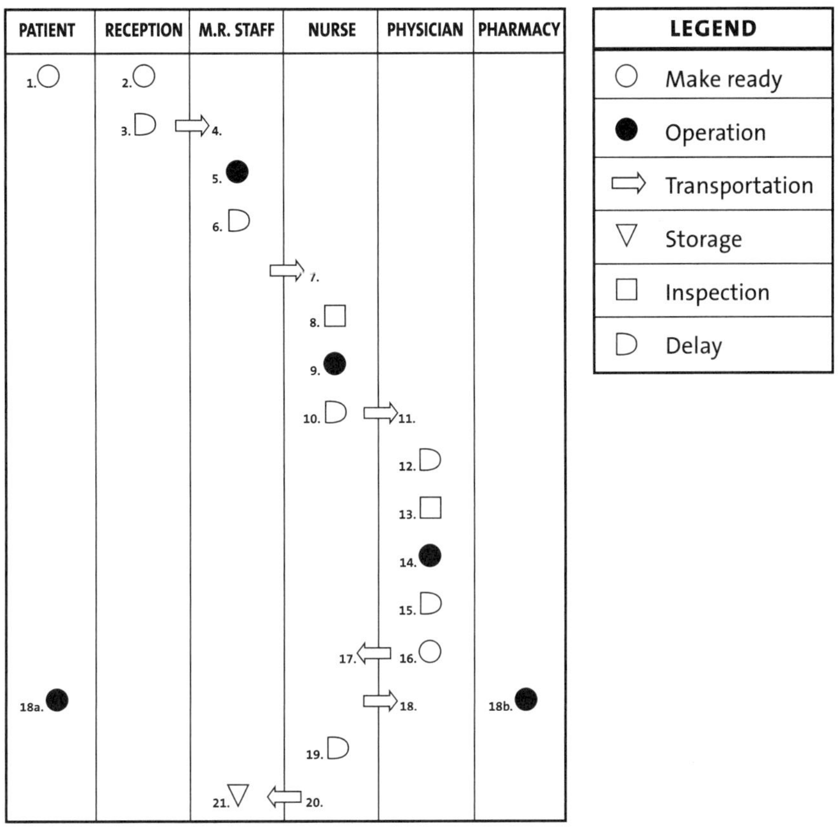

Reprinted with permission, Margret\A Consulting, LLC

the screen without special instruction or memorizing various pathway directions?

▶ *Use of color, icons, and animation.* This refers to how various aids help users to be aware of alerts and reminders or the status of various information. Color is commonly used to highlight items needing attention, such as when something must be signed, when there is an abnormal lab result, when the code does not match the documentation, or when there is new information. Be aware, however, that many people, primarily males, are color-blind, and the amount of ambient light in a room can distort gradations in color, so color is sometimes unreliable as an indicator. Icons are intended to provide quick information as to what can be accomplished by certain actions. Many common icons are in use. For example, a file folder icon may be used to indicate that a record is open or can be saved, scissors can denote that data can be cut, and two documents can denote that data can be copied. Icons can be effective in making screens intuitive, but they must be large enough to discern and be commonly applied. Animation is often coupled with color to highlight an alert or reminder. Be aware, however, that too much color, icon usage, and animation can be distracting and irritating.

▶ *Structured data entry techniques.* This refers to aids used to help enter data. Structured templates provide for the ability to enter variable data into a pre-designed report. For example, a well-baby template for a pediatric practice can establish all of the items to be recorded. Some structured templates require that variable data be entered using standard vocabulary and therefore may provide drop-down menus or smart text for this purpose. In other cases, the variable data entered may be unstructured. Highly structured templates provide for data entry via checkboxes and/or radio buttons.

▶ *Level of detail.* This refers to the number of screens needing to be accessed to get to information. Level of detail is an important consideration. Most experts suggest that people start to feel they have lost their place in the system if they have to "drill down" more than three layers in total. An EHR that provides for summary and detail information is ideal, but it needs to be carefully managed.

Another process issue is the amount of data captured and retrieved. Because computers can process vast amounts of data virtually instantaneously, there can be a tendency to attempt to capture too much information. Each practice should assess this in light of individual needs, also making sure the system can accommodate additional information needs in the future. A good example of this involves prescription refills. If the provider elects to prescribe an off-formulary drug, some systems allow the prescriber to document and transmit the rationale for this to avoid a potential call from the pharmacist. However, this information is not something that has typically been documented in medical records, and it may not be necessary in the future either.

▶ Special Considerations

A final element in your planning for an EHR should be identifying any special considerations needed for your EHR. These may be related to your specialty, state law, accreditation requirements, or other factors.

For example, a pediatrician may want to make sure the HCI devices in the practice are "kid-proofed," perhaps with plastic covers over keyboards or touch screens. A pediatric practice will also want to be sure that e-prescribing components provide very specific dosing calculations to accommodate children's needs.

Many specialists want templates that are already designed to help them capture the information they especially need. Clearly, a cardiologist will have very different needs from an orthopedic surgeon or a psychiatrist. In addition to specific content for the templates, some of the differences may include the availability of drawing tools, sophisticated picture processing aids, ability to handle streaming video, use of certain standard vocabulary, and so on. Some vendors have a wide range of clinical specialty templates; others are more primary-care oriented. In addition, some vendors have designed their products with an emphasis on other aspects of specialty care. Another consideration is data reporting requirements. For example, community health centers have highly regulated requirements, and managed care practices have unique data requirements. It is worth shopping around, depending on the nature of your practice and future plans.

State law has generally been very supportive of EHR systems, but certain states still require wet signatures or formats of prescriptions, especially for controlled substances. Check with your state medical society and/or legal counsel on this issue before making a final vendor decision.

More and more practices are starting to look at Joint Commission on Accreditation of Healthcare Organization (JCAHO) or other accreditation. Although many such organizations are generally very supportive of EHR system use, there may be special requirements to highlight in your selection process.

▶ Conclusion

Perhaps the most important advice to bear in mind as you approach vendor selection is that everyone in the practice who will use the system in some way needs to be engaged in the evaluation to get a well-rounded perspective. If the system works for some but not for others in the practice, there will always be tensions, bottlenecks, and workarounds that limit the value of the system.

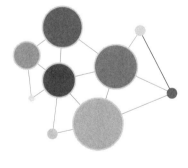

SIX

How to Select the Right Vendor and EHR for Your Practice

Selecting the right vendor solution(s) for your practice is a multi-step process. Each of the steps are designed to consistently identify and focus on the objectives and business needs of your organization from an overall practice perspective. This is a valuable concept for the project leader and EHR team to understand and follow to ensure a match between the solutions selected and the resources and requirements of your organization.

THIS CHAPTER HELPS you:

- ► Understand the process for using your practice's functional needs;

- ► Save time and resources by identifying and focusing on your practice's specific requirements;

- ► Obtain a clear reading of your executive management's commitment to moving forward with system selection and implementation;

- ► Construct a budget for EHR implementation and ongoing operations;

- ► Develop a process that focuses your resources and decision making on your practice's priorities;

- ► Prepare a request for proposal (RFP) to solicit responses from appropriate vendors; and

▶ Select a vendor that meets your requirements and will meet your future needs.

▶ The Importance of Selecting the Right Vendor and EHR for your Practice

Group practices have many common characteristics. Most, however, also have unique aspects, including the practice's style, its work flow preferences, and the degree to which the practice interrelates with other providers or is primarily self contained to provide patient care. When selecting a vendor and application for a particular practice, all too often the administrator asks other administrators in the same specialty for recommendations. Some practices consult a commercial service that rates vendor products as their primary mechanism to select a vendor. Although some useful information may be gathered from these research efforts, they are not the best means to select the right vendor and application. The most important reasons that you should not rely entirely on these types of sources are:

▶ The information system (IS) requirements of the other administrators and the perspectives of the respondents for the rating surveys may be different from yours.

▶ You are conducting a search and selection process based on current product availability, whereas the colleagues you are asking are responding for products that they might have installed a while ago, some of which may not even be currently available.

The following posting on the MGMA Information Management Society (IMS) e-mail forum on July 27, 2004, shows such an indiscriminate solicitation: "Hello everyone, Has anyone ever heard of (good or bad or really bad) about vendor XXX? Thanks in advance." You should be more discriminating about whom you are asking for a reference.

Vendors (and applications) that rate high through references and ratings based on practice situations similar to yours should be considered, but a low ranking or absence from a reference may not be important to your search. Instead, you should base your selection criteria primarily on the specific requirements of your practice. This will help you focus on the vendors and applications that can best support your needs based on the process described in Chapter 5, Determining and Managing Your Requirements.

▶ Practice Leadership Approval and Commitment

In the past, medical practice leadership – administrator, chief financial officer (CFO), chief operating officer (COO), and physician president – and the board of directors were involved in IS primarily from a budget perspective. The billing system, transcription/word processing, and network infrastructure were technology automation capabilities that were used primarily by medical records, registration, appointment scheduling, and billing personnel. To the extent that the appointment schedule was managed and supported centrally, the physician's day-to-day practice was impacted by policies and procedures regarding the schedule, such as the number of days off, vacation schedule, and the need to have the appropriate number of physicians in the practice each day. But all of the other IS applications were invisible to the physician in the daily treatment of patients.

With the implementation of an EHR, all clinicians in the practice and most non-clinical staff are directly impacted in their everyday activities to the extent that data flows and work flows are automated. Some changes impact only an individual physician's treatment of a specific patient. For example, consider an EHR application that has treatment documentation integrated with a function that validates the appropriateness of the documented procedure codes used for billing with the documented diagnosis and treatment in the record. Then the rules that are established by the practice on what happens when the documentation is inconsistent with the procedure and/or diagnoses codes could impact the physician, ranging from complete override capability with minimal impact on the physician to utilizing a forced change in documentation or the procedure/diagnosis information to assure compatibility.

The effective use of an EHR in a physician group practice depends on a change in the practice's culture and adoption of work flow standards to achieve improvements in patient care, accurate and complete billing, and increased productivity. Time should be set aside for physicians and other clinician champions to participate in the design and training functions. The information technology (IT) capital investment and ongoing staffing and maintenance costs will therefore be higher than current expenditure levels. These increased costs can be offset through staff reassignments and reductions, as well as increased productivity.[1]

The leadership of the practice as well as the board must approve the new direction as well as provide leadership support and commitment to make the change successful. Therefore, use one or more of the following tools to provide a picture of the expected costs, benefits, processes, and barriers to the leadership or final decision makers:

- ▶ A high-level project plan complete with timelines, including system selection, equipment acquisition and testing, data conversion, new EHR system implementation, and phase-out of legacy applications;

- ▶ A list of the proposed project team members and the roles of physicians and other clinician leaders in the process;

- ▶ A draft budget with an approximate timeline as to when the expenditures will occur;

- ▶ A list of key goals and benefits; and

- ▶ A summary of the process undertaken to date, including the development of your group practice's requirements.

When the practice leadership has approved the plan and committed to it, you are ready to move forward with selecting and implementing an EHR. Periodic reporting to those in authority, as well as regular updates to the entire staff are strongly recommended. To protect the interests of the practice, limit the specific details on vendors and the selection process, evaluation scores, and cost information to a small group of individuals directly involved in the selection process. However, you should require non-confidentiality for the vendor proposals and demonstrations, except for pricing data, so that you are able to freely use the information in the evaluation process. Materials submitted by vendors and staff notes that are no longer needed should be kept in a secure place under the control of the project manager. Sixty days (or a longer period consistent with your record policies or legal advice) after the completion of successful contract negotiations, destroy all vendor-supplied documents and evaluation materials, except those for the selected vendor and the second-place vendor (just in case you need to change vendors.) Vendors may allege that proposals contain some proprietary information, so it is best to destroy these unneeded documents.

▶ Selecting the Vendor Candidates That Best Match Your Requirements

At least two approaches exist for finding an IS vendor and EHR that best suit your needs. The two approaches differ primarily in the number of candidates that receive the RFP.

Some organizations take the "shotgun" approach, sending their RFPs to every vendor candidate they can identify. On the surface, this sounds like an efficient approach, even if you can obtain a list of 50 or more EHR vendors. However, it is not a very productive approach. At this early stage of the selection process, the goal is to identify three to six vendors that will most likely meet your requirements. To do this, you need to obtain responses to your RFP (discussed in the next section) from those top candidates. If the invitation to bid is sent to 50-plus companies, most vendors will either not be interested in responding at all or will respond only with generic marketing information or a proposal prepared by an RFP-automated response tool. With such a shotgun approach, you could miss the best candidates to meet your needs, or you could be overwhelmed with information, at lot of which is not useful.

The recommended approach is to identify a list of 8 to 15 vendor candidates to evaluate for their ability to meet your requirements. One way to obtain such a candidate list is to use a consultant service that has information on the functional capabilities of the EHR vendor products. Some interpretation will be required because physician practice EHR vendors do not use standard terminology to categorize functional requirements, although this may change through the use of the Health Level Seven® (HL7®) EHR functional description adopted for trial use in 2004.[2] You can also obtain some information about vendor products at individual vendor Web sites. In addition, check the Web sites of market research and analysis firms specializing in medical information systems, such as Jewson Enterprises,[3] KLAS,[4] as well as MGMA affiliates and exhibitors.

The remaining sections of this chapter discuss a business approach to selecting your EHR vendor through a series of steps that systematically reduces the number of candidates by learning additional information on each remaining candidate and adjusting the evaluation scores based on the additional information. The steps in the example used in this chapter are:

1. From EHR lists and general information vendors, identify 8 to 15 vendor candidates;

2. Based on your requirements, EHR vendor marketing material, consultants, and references, select three to six vendors to receive your RFP;

3. After proposal and demonstration evaluations, select the top two to four vendors for additional questions and references;

4. Next, conduct site visits to the top two or three vendor client sites; and

5. Prioritize the finalists and negotiate with the top vendor (or top two if the rankings are very close).

▶ Obtaining Value from the Formal RFP Process

Most health care organizations approach an EHR selection process in one of two ways. One approach involves first defining your practice's requirements and then including these requirements with other specifications in a written RFP. The second, less formal process involves inviting multiple vendors to conduct demonstrations at your organization. Then individuals review what they have seen and either make a final selection or significantly narrow the field and base the vendor selection primarily on the demonstrations.

Pros and cons are associated with either approach, as summarized in Exhibits 6.1 and 6.2 for the structured RFP approach and the vendor demon-

---

EXHIBIT 6.1 Structured RFP Approach 0100101001000010001100

PRO

- ▶ Provides an excellent opportunity to identify and quantify your practice's requirements;
- ▶ Offers a structured basis for scoring vendor products based on your priorities;
- ▶ Allows you to receive information and simultaneously evaluate important factors besides functionality, including:
  - ▷ Cost
  - ▷ Service and support commitment
  - ▷ Vendor financial stability
  - ▷ Willingness to commit to your requirements in writing;
- ▶ Results in fewer demonstrations – the RFP responses can be used to select the smaller pool of vendors that will be invited to demonstrate in your practice;
- ▶ Saves clinicians' time by having them view fewer demonstrations after the proposal review; and
- ▶ Saves clinician time by focusing clinician evaluations/observations on those products most likely to meet your functional and business needs.

CON

- ▶ May be difficult to articulate and reach agreement on your business needs; and
- ▶ Takes dedicated time to write the RFP.

Reprinted with permission, Boundary Information Group

EXHIBIT 6.2   Vendor Demonstration as the Primary Selection Process

PRO

- ▶ Allows you to observe live demonstrations of functionality;
- ▶ Provides the opportunity to create a functional vision for clinicians and others;
- ▶ Can include role playing; and
- ▶ Can show how data flow and work flow are related in a demonstration mode.

CON

- ▶ Takes a lot of your staff time (1-2 hours per attendee per demonstration);
- ▶ Focuses on what the vendor wants to show, not on what you need to see (unless you require a demonstration to your script/scenario specification);
- ▶ May not provide useful information – all vendors worth consideration can present a good demonstration, but that may not translate into the appropriate product for your practice;
- ▶ May be misleading – preloaded responses and small files can result in a positive demonstration that makes the system look simpler and/or faster to use than it really is; and
- ▶ May influence evaluation scores more by the demonstrator/salesperson team than by the system capabilities (unless you train your observers well).

Reprinted with permission, Boundary Information Group

stration, respectively. Most organizations will find that the formal RFP process reduces the risk of a failed project and increases the likelihood that the resulting EHR selection implementation is a good fit with the organization's clinical and business needs. It also has the tendency to lower the overall cost because it includes the specification of all of the components that you will need to complete and support the implementation. For instance, the RFP pricing section should require the bidder to list the prices for training, installation support, interfaces, travel, databases (e.g., CPT®, drug formulary). A vendor proposal based on demonstrations may not include the customer's specification list.

▶ In-House vs. Application Service Provider Solutions

Two technology strategies exist for your EHR. With either strategy, your organization will be licensing the EHR application, although the financial arrangements and term of license options may be different with each strategy.

One choice is to locate and maintain all the hardware, operating systems, and EHR applications in a facility that you own or lease, supported by your staff (perhaps with outside contractor's support). This is sometimes referred to as an in-house solution. An alternative is to have the EHR vendor, or a third party, host the application in its facility on hardware that either you or the vendor owns, with your staff operating the EHR. If data communication to the host is over the Internet, this latter strategy is referred to as an application service provider (ASP) solution. If the data communication is over telephone lines or frame relay, it may be called remote hosting.

Mid-sized to large group practices will almost always find it financially attractive to maintain the hardware and software in-house, along with having their own staffs provide all or most of the technical support services. For smaller physician practices, or physician practices in rural areas where access to technical personnel may be limited, the ASP option is worth considering. Physicians near retirement and young physicians who lack capital or credit access may benefit from the ASP subscription model.[5] Some of the primary differences between in-house and ASP solutions are summarized in Exhibit 6.3.

▶ EHR Integration/Interfacing with PMS – Does It Matter?

Your EHR must be able to communicate electronic data back and forth with your PMS. This can be accomplished in at least three different ways. The first two are variations of EHR-PMS integration, which means that the data and functionality are integrated between the two applications. The third, an EHR-PMS interface, views the applications as two databases and two separate applications without integrated functionality.

EHR-PMS Integration with a Common Data Dictionary and Functionality

Integration can be accomplished with a partial common database and compatible functionality between the EHR and the PMS. Usually this is accomplished by having a single vendor solution with EHR and PMS product offerings that have been designed to integrate functionally with a common database or with two databases that are automatically synchronized. For instance, the PMS database and the clinical data repository in the EHR can have a common data dictionary and tools to synchronize data transfer between the two. Examples of how this integration works are the following:

EXHIBIT 6.3   ASP vs. In-House EHR   1001010010100100001000110

EHR CHARACTERISTICS	ASP	IN-HOUSE
Secure data center	Usually available; usually designed to meet many of your HIPAA Security Rule requirements.	You are responsible for building and maintaining a data center that is secure.
Technical staff	ASP vendor provides around-the-clock (24/7) technical staff support to maintain and support servers, operating systems, and perhaps the application.	You must provide technical support for the servers, operating systems and application for at least the hours of your business operations (24/7 support is recommended because if the server goes down in the middle of the night, it must be restored for clinicians to see patients the next morning during normal office hours).
Help desk	May supply 24/7 help desk for server, operating system, password, and basic functionality.	Your staff must provide 24/7 support (or at least for all hours of your operation).
Customized EHR functionality	Customized EHR functionality support is provided for your organization.	Customized EHR functionality support is provided by your organization.
Cost	Cost could vary, depending on many factors.[6] Potential areas of cost savings are shared technical support staff over many ASP customers, shared cost of security technology among ASP customers, and volume discounts for servers and backup technology available to the ASP due to its large customer base. Secured data communication costs from your location to the ASP host could be a factor, depending on circumstances and the technology used.	Cost varies by size of practice and level of service.

Reprinted with Permission, Boundary Information Group

▶ Recording or changing the patient's phone number can be accomplished in either the registration system (part of the PMS) or the collection of vital signs and information in an initial interview as part of an office visit (part of the EHR). It doesn't matter where it occurs because the data are maintained in the same database and are accessible to both applications.

▶ The next appointment can be scheduled through the EHR as part of the physician's completion of the office visit, or it can be handled through the checkout desk or reception desk through the PMS. All users could be set up to have access to appointment scheduling based on the work flow required by the practice. Because the applications and database are integrated, the practice can decide how it wants the appointment scheduling work flow to occur for follow-up appointments. This seamless functionality may be truly integrated into a combined EHR/PMS application that is fully integrated, or the functionality/access can be integrated in such a way that, although the appointment scheduling module is part of the PMS, its access is fully integrated into the EHR, and to the EHR user it appears as part of the EHR.

EHR-PMS Integration: Separate Databases

In some cases, EHR vendors have partially integrated solutions with their own PMSs or other products. Often, the accounts receivable database for the PMS and the accounts in the clinical data repository for the EHR are separate, but a mechanism is used to integrate the patient demographics so that, for example, the phone number change presented in the first example above is functionally integrated, but the appointment scheduling functionality is maintained in either the PMS or the EHR. Access can be provided to the appointment scheduling module from the non-hosting system by clicking on an icon, and the application will have the look and feel of the hosting application, which may be different from the screen used to access appointment scheduling through an icon. In those cases for which the same vendor has supplied both the PMS and EHR, the look and feel may be the same for both and the user will not be aware of the difference. The integrated access process will transfer the patient demographic data to the other application automatically, so no re-keying of patient name or other data is necessary.

The technology infrastructure to support this approach is different from an integrated solution with a common database. The PMS and EHR are on two separate databases, usually hosted on two separate servers, and they may have technologically different database platforms from different vendors.

This multiple database structure has significant implications for report writing and data dictionary management. Through the use of third-party report-writing tools, such as Crystal Reports™, however, some of these differences can be addressed without significant difficulty or cost. Each combination of vendors needs to be assessed based on the parameters involved to determine whether this is a significant issue that will be difficult to address or one that is easily accommodated. Usually, the cost is higher for this option due to the additional hardware database licenses and user licenses involved. Again, each vendor offering needs to be evaluated based on the specifics proposed and requirements of your practice.

EHR and PMS Interfaced Solution

An EHR and PMS interface means that the data captured and recorded in one system is transferred to the other system through an electronic data interface. Often, with EHR and PMS applications, a two-way interface is required. Because data transmission delays are often associated with interfacing (which could be in a batch mode periodically or in real time), functions such as validating procedure coding with documentation through the PMS may not be feasible while the physician is still working with the EHR patient documentation. Usually in this structure, the two databases for the PMS and EHR have to be updated separately and potentially could have different data element values at any specific time.

Many physician practices have a PMS that functions well for them and is in the earlier phases of its life cycle. If this is the case for your practice, diligently review of the options, costs, and benefits of (1) having an interfaced solution with the PMS, (2) utilizing an integrated EHR offered by the PMS vendor or another EHR vendor that meets your practice EHR requirements, or (3) replacing your PMS with a new one as part of the process of implementing the EHR so that you have functional and data integration of the PMS and the EHR. For older PMS applications, functional limitations and the challenges of interfacing may exclude a practical option of continuing the use of the current PMS.

▶ Managing the Competitive Bid, Evaluation, and Selection Process

A significant amount of work is associated with managing the process, from specifying your practice's requirements for an EHR to completing the selection of an EHR (and perhaps a PMS) product. The work becomes more intense during the preparation for and implementation of the EHR. Resources and project management skills are needed to successfully keep this process on track and focused on the project goals.

A project manager should be appointed to manage this process. The competitive bid and selection process will take several months – six to nine months is a realistic time range for the process based on the steps outlined in Exhibit 6.4; use this template to establish your timeline.

The system selection process is best conducted as a structured one, with objective criteria used to the greatest extent possible. This accomplishes several objectives that are important to your practice.

- ▶ It keeps the process moving along consistent with your milestones, so you accomplish the task in a reasonable time. The vendors will continue to have an interest in you, especially as the number of vendor candidates left in the process decreases.

- ▶ Objectivity rather than subjectivity will drive the ranking of the vendors toward your practice's requirements and criteria. Subjective evaluations tend to give unwarranted weight to the best demonstration, the best brochures, the lowest cost and/or the vendor customer base, or to some function that is not part of your important requirements that they perform very well.

- ▶ A structured process almost always results in a relatively quick narrowing of the field of candidate vendors to only those that best meet your requirements.

Experience in information systems selection for medical groups and other organizations has determined that the following general principles will protect the assets of your group:

- ▶ Once the RFP has been issued, no new vendors should be admitted into the process. Exhibit 6.5 on page 159 presents sample contents of an RFP. The RFP is very important in that it tells the vendors what you are looking for and provides a consistent format structure for their proposals, which will help in your evaluation. This document, together with the vendor's proposal and other vendor documents, will become part of the contract you eventually negotiate with the selected vendor.

- ▶ Only the evaluation committee should receive and review the proposals. Internal or external consultants can be used for a focused review of a specific aspect of the proposal, such as a

EXHIBIT 6.4 Steps for the Vendor Selection Process 0001000110

ACTIVITY	TIME FRAME
1. Identify the EHR selection project manager and committee, and allocate time devoted to the project.	
2. Develop a written RFP based on your requirements.	
3. Identify the list of vendors who will receive the RFP.	
4. Develop a timeline for each of the remaining steps in the system selection process.	
5. Assemble and issue the RFP to the selected vendors.	
6. Identify the person to receive all communications and proposals from the vendors in response to the RFP and follow-up (this person may be the project manager).	
7. Develop the proposal evaluation tools, criteria, and evaluation team.	
8. Arrange for vendor site visits to your facility to review your business needs.	
9. Include EHR vendor product demonstrations as part of the site visits.	
10. Evaluate proposals.	
11. Develop additional questions for the top two to four vendors.	
12. Check references of the top two to four vendors.	
13. Update the evaluations based on references and answers to questions.	
14. Narrow the selection to the top two or three vendors.	
15. Develop tools for evaluating site visits.	
16. Schedule site visits to vendor customers and headquarters.	
17. If needed, ask vendors additional questions or clarifications in writing, and receive the written responses.	
18. Select the final two vendors (or three, if warranted due to close results) with priority ranking.	

continued next page

EXHIBIT 6.4   Steps for the Vendor Selection Process *continued*

ACTIVITY	TIME FRAME
19. Seek internal approval and proceed with negotiations; if the expected cost is outside the approved budget, seek additional budget approval or reduce scope/capability.	
20. Negotiate contract with first-choice vendor.	
21. Successfully conclude negotiations.	

Reprinted with permission, Boundary Information Group

proposed technology that the committee does not have the expertise to evaluate.

▶ Reference calls and site visits should, to the greatest extent possible, be undertaken with organizations of your same size and specialty. If you are integrating or interfacing the EHR to a PMS, consider only those with the same PMS product you are proposing to use.

▶ The reference calls and site visits should be planned with specific questions and issues to be addressed. Listen carefully and observe the attitudes of the users.

▶ As part of the vendor user site visits, you should require a private interview (a half hour or more) with a customer executive without the vendor being present. Interview questions should be focused on leadership satisfaction with the EHR in supporting the organization's goals and internal staff requirements, as well as advice on how to be successful.

▶ Physician and non-physician clinician leaders must participate in the demonstrations at your facility and in the site visits so that your practice is assured that the clinicians' interests are being well represented in the process. Exhibit 6.6 on page 160 outlines the steps for conducting an objective vendor demonstration. Remember, you set the rules for the demonstration so that your staff time is best utilized in observing functionality and your questions are addressed.[7]

▶ Clinicians' interests need to be included directly in the evaluation team.

▶ Negotiations for the contract are often about more than the cost. They may include service level agreements, delivery dates, assurances of conversion of existing data, and so forth. The overall cost analysis should include staff time, travel for training, hardware that you will purchase directly, and interface programming and testing with the applications. In your negotiations, remember that it is always good to get a lower price, but the vendor has to make enough money to stay in business.

EXHIBIT 6.5   Example of RFP Contents   0100010100100001000110

1. Purpose of RFP
2. Timeline for key steps in the selection process
   ▶ Issue RFP
   ▶ Dates for site visit/interview/demonstrations at your location
   ▶ Proposal due date
   ▶ Target selection completion date
3. Contact information
4. Number of copies and delivery location; whether submissions are to be paper or electronic
5. Format and guidelines for the proposal to be addressed by vendor
   ▶ Vendor capabilities for your specific functional requirements
   ▶ Company (vendor's) information
     ▷ Financial information
     ▷ Background
     ▷ Commitment to the proposed application
     ▷ Customer references
   ▶ Technical and cost format instructions
   ▶ Your terms and conditions

Reprinted with permission, Boundary Information Group

▶ Reference Checking and Site Visits

Reference checking and site visits are two important data-gathering steps in the system selection process. Both involve the use of vendor customers' valuable time, so these important processes for information gathering should be limited to your finalist vendors (no more than four), and to the greatest extent possible they should focus on installations with the same version of the product that you are considering and an environment as similar to your own practice as possible.

EXHIBIT 6.6   Steps for Conducting Objective Vendor Demonstrations

1. You control the agenda:
   ▶ Limit company background and introduction to five minutes;
   ▶ Tell the vendor in writing what you want demonstrated; and
   ▶ Let demonstration attendees ask questions, but give priority to answers that demonstrate the application. Many questions (e.g., who are your customers?) can be answered later.

2. Orient your staff on the purpose of the demonstration, what to expect, and your evaluation procedure.

3. Use a one-page evaluation form to obtain feedback from all demonstration attendees.

4. Collect the completed evaluation forms before the observers leave the demonstration.

5. Keep on schedule – your staff's time is valuable.

6. Urge the vendors to test their demonstration at your site before the scheduled start time so that everything works and there are no delays.

Reprinted with permission, Boundary Information Group

Reference Checking

Reference checking can be performed before or after the proposal evaluation process narrows the field to the top two or four vendors that meet your requirements. Ask vendors which references in their proposals meet the criterion of same product installation in organizations similar to your own, and feel free to call other individuals at those reference sites as well. Also contact users of the product who are known to you and are not on the vendor's reference list. For this latter group, make sure that they are using the same version and applications of the product as the one you are considering. Ask whether there is an active user group and what value you will gain from it.

Exhibit 6.7 lists questions that can be included in the reference telephone interview. Usually, reference checking is done by telephone by two or three members of your evaluation team. (More than one person should conduct the reference interviews to minimize the chance for bias.) Have the same two or three people conduct all of the reference interviews to assure consistency. Typically, two or three reference interviews are conducted per vendor. The interviews should follow a structured format to assure that all of your reference questions are answered. Part of the interview process is to document the answers to the questions and share those with the evaluation committee.

It is a nice touch to send a note or e-mail to the references after you have completed the interviews, thanking them for their time and honesty.

EXHIBIT 6.7 Reference Interview Questions 1010010000100011001

1. How would you describe your organization in terms of number of physicians, specialty mix, and number of sites?

2. What is the current version of the (vendor's) product that you have installed? When did it go live?

3. What do you like most about the product?

4. What other primary information system products, either from this vendor or others, have been installed in your organization?

5. What type of team do you have on an ongoing basis to maintain and enhance the use of the application?

6. What interfaces do you have to and from this application to other systems applications from different vendors?

7. Is the application deployed throughout your whole enterprise or only in some settings?

8. What types of end-user devices do you use with the application (for example, desktop, notepad, PC tablet, PDA)?

9. How long does it take physicians to learn how to use the system with full competency?

10. What training methods did you use for physicians and other clinicians to successfully get them into a productive mode quickly?

11. How would you describe your implementation team, process, and length of time for the EHR?

12. What does your organization like best about the EHR?

13. What does your organization like least about the EHR? What poses the most problems?

14. If you had to do the implementation over again, what would you do differently?

15. What savings have you achieved with the implementation of the EHR, and how did you go about achieving them?

16. Is there an enhancement to the EHR that the vendor has been promising but has not delivered, which we could include as a contractual condition that would also benefit you?

17. May we have the name and phone number of your CFO and your administrator, and is it okay if our CFO and administrator contact them?

18. Is there anything else that you would like to tell us about your experience with the EHR product?

Reprinted with permission, Boundary Information Group

Site Visits

Site visits are an important investigative methodology during the evaluation process. They are expensive for you, for the vendor, and for the vendor user that you visit, so they should be limited to your two top finalist vendors. It is common to conduct two site visits per vendor, with a team of individuals from your organization representing all of the key operational components of your EHR implementation. As an option, include the vendor headquarters as a third site. Examples of the types of representatives to include on a site-visit team are presented in Exhibit 6.8. All of your administrative, technical, and clinical components should be represented on each site visit.

Site visit pros and cons are summarized in Exhibit 6.9. Site visits (and reference checks) can satisfy two objectives. The primary one is to evaluate the EHR vendor's product implementation in an environment similar to yours. A site visit can validate whether the system works as the vendor says it does in the proposal and can help determine the resources that are needed to support the product on an ongoing basis in an environment similar to

EXHIBIT 6.8 Composition of the Site Visit Team 0100001000011100

ROLE	YOUR PRACTICE'S PARTICIPANTS
Administrator/Chief financial officer	
Manager/Chief operating officer	
Clinic operations	
Physician	
Nurse/Physician's assistant	
EHR Project manager	
Medical records/Health information management	
Chief information officer/IT director	
Database administrator and/or Server IT staff	
Health data analyst/Report administrator	
EHR selection consultants	

Reprinted with permission, Boundary Information Group

EXHIBIT 6.9 Site Visits as Part of the Selection Process 0001100

PRO

Site visits provide an opportunity to:

▶ Observe live use of the EHR functionality;

▶ See other physicians using the EHR and the changes in work flow to support the use (especially helpful to your own physicians);

▶ Understand technical support requirements and staffing based on use;

▶ Evaluate the effectiveness of interfaces to PMS and other applications if they are the same as yours; and

▶ Visualize the needed changes in work flow (especially important to clinicians).

CON

Site visits can:

▶ Take a lot of staff time (additionally, clinicians may lose production); and

▶ Be conducted at a practice that is not very similar to yours.

Reprinted with permission, Boundary Information Group

yours. The second objective is to understand the work flow and other changes that were implemented to achieve significant benefits from the EHR. All site visits where there are successful EHR implementations, regardless of whether they use the vendor's application that you finally select, can supply valuable information to your team.

▶ The Process of Moving from Many Vendors to One Vendor

For all of the proposals remaining active in the selection process at this point, you should have completed the following steps:

1. Receive and evaluate each bidder's proposal;

2. Conduct and document demonstration evaluations;

3. Conduct and document reference checks; and

4. Ask and receive written answers to specific questions that you asked the vendor based on the proposal and other information.

The task now is to rank the final two (or three, if warranted due to close results) vendors that are a good fit for the organization from the remaining

001010010110100101001010010100

An Example of Physician Leadership

A hospital with a significant ambulatory care operation including several employed physicians was faced with the decision of selecting one of two finalist EHR vendors as the winner. A dozen physicians and nurses had accompanied the EHR Steering Committee on the two final one-day site visits, one for each vendor. They all met the morning after the second site visit to make the recommendation. All of the participants knew that one of the EHR vendor's costs were a lot higher than the other, but specific pricing details had not been disclosed to them. After 30 minutes of expressing obvious pros and cons, one of the physician leaders stood up and said, "One of these vendors presents us with the future and supports how we want to practice using an electronic health record system. The other presents us with an automation of our paper processes that we know are broken. Either way we are going to invest a lot of money and time in moving from where we are to one of these two vendor products. Strategically, we should move to the solution that moves us to the future. Even though it will be harder for us to make the transition, it will take us to where we need to go."

Thus the organization decided to move forward with an EHR that supported new work flows and an integrated enterprise solution that would significantly change the culture of the organization and greatly enhance its ability to provide quality care to patients.

vendors. At this point, if necessary, have the vendors commit to changing their proposals to more favorably reflect your business needs.

Sometimes the process of ranking the final vendors is easy. Perhaps one is far superior on performance to the other(s), and they have comparable cost (see the next section, Constructing a Budget for EHR). Sometimes the functional capabilities and support for the organization seem equal (and ranked high), but there is a big difference in cost. A more difficult challenge is presented when one of the remaining vendors is high on performance and high on cost, and the other is lower on performance (barely acceptable) and low on cost. It is important to select the vendor that will work long-term with your organization to meet your current business requirements and anticipated future requirements at a cost that is affordable. The finalist should offer a reasonable return on investment (ROI), improve work processes, and support quality of care for your practice.

Because the physicians and other clinicians in your practice will be the primary users of the EHR, their opinions must be weighed significantly in the final selection process. If the evaluation results are extremely close between two finalists, negotiate with both of them. Even if you decide that there is a clear winner, do not let either vendor know there is only one left. You will be in a much stronger negotiating position if the winning vendor doesn't know it is the only one left.

▶ Constructing a Budget for EHR

It is important to construct a budget for the EHR that includes direct and indirect costs associated with the EHR products and services, EHR support and infrastructure changes, and ongoing expenses (including maintenance fees and staff). This budget should also reflect savings that are expected to occur after the initial implementation. These savings may be reflected in the budget itself or as notes so that the net financial outlay is understood by practice leadership and the board. Refer to the discussion in Chapter 4, Return on Investment, for the ROI cost worksheet example. The budget developed at this stage can reflect specifics based on the vendor finalist proposal(s) and your plans for implementation and operations.

The planning, selection, implementation, and operations of the EHR span several years, so a multi-year budget approach (a minimum of three years) is highly recommended. If your medical group is accustomed to financing software and hardware with a multi-year payoff, you should also create a version of the budget that lasts as long as the payoff period. An alternative management version of the budget could reflect a shorter time period, such as the three-year period reflected in Exhibit 6.10 on pages 166–67. Another planning tool for EMR budgeting is available on the Internet from the American Academy of Family Practice.[8]

The first year of the budget should reflect the costs associated with planning for the EHR (and PMS, if involved in the same project). This includes collecting background information, organizing a project team, developing the requirements analysis/strategic objectives of the organization, researching potential vendors and infrastructure options, and preparing the RFP and the selection process. Early stages of the implementation may also be included in the first year, depending on how rapidly the organization proceeds through this process. Typically, a medical group practice will spend 6 to 12 months from the beginning of researching the EHR initiative to selecting a system. An even longer time frame (15 to 18 months) can occur in special circumstances, such as an EHR initiative and overall IT restructuring being designed to bring two organizations under one IS infrastructure and set of applications in the case of a merger.

EXHIBIT 6.10 Budget Template 0110100101001010010000010001100

ITEMS	BUDGET ESTIMATE		
	YEAR 1 $	YEAR 2 $	YEAR 3 $
1. EHR Software Additional Software ▶ Interfaces ▶ Report writer ▶ Database ▶ Microsoft Office® ▶ PC operating system ▶ Server operating system ▶ Other			
2. Hardware ▶ Servers ▶ User workstations/devices ▶ Other			
3. Network/Infrastructure enhancement ▶ Backup/archiving ▶ Single sign-on ▶ Mirrored processing ▶ (Redundant) data communications among sites ▶ Wireless ▶ Other			
4. Data (Electronic) ▶ Drug formularies ▶ Drug reference information (e.g., *Physicians' Desk Reference®*) ▶ Patient education ▶ Other			
5. Data Communications Management ▶ EHR e-prescribing ▶ Other			
6. Vendor Installation Support ▶ Initial hardware and software installation ▶ Software customization management ▶ Software updates ▶ Training ▶ Data conversion ▶ Customized interfaces and testing ▶ Other			

EXHIBIT 6.10 **Budget Template** *continued* 100101001000010001100

ITEMS	BUDGET ESTIMATE		
	YEAR 1 $	YEAR 2 $	YEAR 3 $
7. Staff			
▶ IT			
▶ User support			
▶ Help desk			
▶ Servers and database			
▶ Manage updates			
▶ Health data analyst/database administrator			
▶ EHR project management			
▶ EHR application analyst(s)			
▶ Training			
▶ Data conversion			
▶ User meeting travel and registration			
▶ Books, subscription services, EHR professional activities, etc.			
▶ Other			
8. Other Services			
▶ EHR consultants			
▶ Off-site disaster recovery location			
▶ Sales tax and shipping			
▶ Other			
9. Contingency Budget (10% of subtotal)			
TOTAL BUDGET			

Reprinted with permission, Boundary Information Group

For most medical groups, the costs of software and hardware acquisition and implementation, plus staff and consultant time associated with implementation and training, will span years 1 and 2. Maintenance cost, ongoing staff support, budget allocation for periodic upgrades, and hardware replacements and/or expansions will be ongoing starting in year 2.

All organizations implementing EHRs will need to review and evaluate their technical infrastructure prior to implementation. This includes IT staff support, data communications/telecommunications (internal and external), hardware (servers, individual handheld and workstation units), licenses (including operating systems and applications), and technology infrastructure (e.g., security, wireless, backup/redundancy, disaster recovery, network management, access control management). Some organizations choose to enhance the technical infrastructure prior to completing the selection of the EHR vendor. Most, however, plan and budget for this process while the EHR planning and vendor selection take place, but wait until the vendor selection is completed before implementing some aspects of the infrastructure to assure it conforms to the requirements of the vendor application selected.

Depending on the number of locations, available staff, and scope of the infrastructure development, implementing the technical infrastructure for the EHR can take several months to more than half a year. Include this cost and timing in the budget process. Recognize, though, that other areas of the practice, in addition to the EHR, will benefit from the enhanced infrastructure.

The budget template items in Exhibit 6.10 are only examples. Your own budget items and cost estimates will be based on your particular situation. When you have progressed through the selection process to the point there are two finalist vendors remaining after evaluating the site visit findings, and you have final proposals with cost estimates from both, it is a good idea to revise your budget based on these estimates.

Some practices are tempted to view the budget for the EHR as being only the cost that they pay the vendor for hardware, software, training time, and implementation support. Although these expenses normally constitute a large portion of the EHR, other components of the budget can be significant. These include staff support, work flow management and analysis, training, data conversion, interface with the PMS, electronic databases to support clinical activities, electronic patient education material, and drug formularies, among others. Often, if these items are not included in the budget, they are not available to the practice when needed, or not to the necessary level, resulting in a less than optimal installation of the EHR. Therefore, be sure your budget is comprehensive, including all costs. In addition, include a 10 percent contingency because unanticipated extra expenses are usually associated with EHR and infrastructure implementation.

By choosing several vendors to bid on your RFP, you place them in a product, service, and cost competitive position. The budget estimate should not be disclosed to potential vendors, nor should the estimated vendor budget be disclosed. You can, however, inform the potential vendors that the organization does have a budget that includes staffing and infrastructure costs beyond expenditures for the vendor. This will encourage many of the vendors to bid on your opportunity because they know you are prepared to support the installation with the resources needed from the practice.

▶ Negotiating the Contract

Contract negotiations began when you wrote your RFP. That document contains the requirements for your organization, your specified terms and conditions, the scope of the procurement, and your required performance criteria. It will become part of the final agreement negotiated between you and the vendor selected for the award.

If you have not already done so prior to this point in the process, form the negotiating team, which in most cases includes two to five individuals from among the following:

- ▶ Administrator or CFO;
- ▶ Legal council;
- ▶ CIO or IT director;
- ▶ EHR consultant; and
- ▶ EHR project manager (ad hoc).

This team will represent your organization in the business of conducting the negotiations to reach a final agreement. It is best not to include the president or board chairman and the administrator in these negotiations so that the negotiating team has the option of reviewing a proposal with "someone with higher authority within the organization" – a useful tactic to allow the negotiating team members to neither refuse nor accept an offer made by the vendor for which they have not had time to give full consideration. In smaller and mid-sized practices, it will often be appropriate to have the administrator directly involved in the negotiations, depending on the skill sets of the other individuals involved. It is very important to have a single spokesperson represent the team in the negotiations. That person can call upon others to elaborate or clarify points that are being made. If a candidate for your negotiating team has a reputation for being independent and speaking his or her mind no matter what the consequences, exclude that person from the negotiations. Your organization's leaders must be comfortable with your team representing them in this important negotiation.

Use legal counsel with experience in drafting and/or negotiating IS contracts. If your internal counsel or general counsel does not have this experience, seek a recommendation from him/her or your EHR consultant. Look for legal counsel with experience in IT contracting and perhaps health care regulatory issues as a secondary capability.

Exhibit 6.11 presents a beginning checklist for negotiations preparation. The agreement that will be reached should incorporate the four types of documentation listed plus additional clauses and exhibits that will assist in performance under the agreement. For instance, you may want to include a payment schedule based on specific milestones.

EXHIBIT 6.11 Negotiations Checklist 0101001010010000010001100

- ❏ Legal support
- ❏ Documentation
  - ❏ Your RFP
  - ❏ Vendor response to RFP
  - ❏ Written questions and answers
  - ❏ Vendors' standard contract(s)
- ❏ Payment schedule based on milestones
- ❏ Criteria for acceptance
- ❏ List of your key issues
- ❏ Clearly defined negotiation authority and team
- ❏ Defined internal approval process

Reprinted with permission, Boundary Information Group

Example milestones for hardware and software payments include the following:

▶ Contract signing;

▶ Delivery, installation, and initial testing of hardware and software;

▶ First productive use in business operations;

▶ Thirty days after first productive use in business operations;

▶ Enterprise-wide productive use; and

▶ XX days after enterprise-wide productive use.

Normally, at least three milestone payments are recommended. For labor that supports implementation, an example payment schedule would be monthly invoices with 90 percent of invoiced and approved labor hours due monthly, and the remainder due on final acceptance and full use of the vendor products.

Tie specific payments to milestones, which should be defined with specific measurable criteria. The first example milestone, "contract signing," is easy to measure. Not more than 25 percent of the total payment of hardware and software should be included with this milestone.

Describe other milestones in detail so the vendor has a clear understanding of the milestone. Milestone 3, "first productive use," should have a measurable definition. For example, it might be one day's patient schedule for one physician or one patient with one physician. It should include all documentation of the diagnosis and treatment for each patient without a separate or supplemental written chart or record, and provide sufficient electronic detail for accurate and timely billing electronically through the PMS without error.

You may also address incentive payments in your negotiations and agreement. Some organizations do fine without incentive contracts. In other cases, vendors and providers find them to be useful. Incentive contracts may be one-sided or bi-directional. One-sided incentive contracts usually are structured so that vendors receive a bonus if the EHR is implemented (per the milestone criteria for full implementation) earlier than expected or on time. Penalties may be imposed on the vendor in the form of reduced price if the full implementation occurs later than stated in the agreement and it is solely the fault of the vendor.

Another approach is to construct an incentive program by which both the vendor and the provider can win or lose financially. The goal is to provide equal incentives for the two organizations to work together for a fully functional, on-time delivery and implementation. This approach should be a consideration for large projects, especially when there is concern on either side that one or more of the parties will have difficulty prioritizing resources to support the project when needed.

Exhibit 6.12 on the next page outlines two incentive alternatives. The first is an incentive program that penalizes the vendor for late delivery and implementation. Because this penalty applies only when the vendor is solely at fault for failure to perform, it can result in a lot of finger pointing and documentation of provider problems. However, this type of program can be an effective way of prioritizing resources from a vendor to focus on your practice's implementation needs to avoid the penalty payment.

Another incentive program, generally used by larger provider organizations, is to structure a mutual bonus and penalty opportunity. This

EXHIBIT 6.12   Examples of Incentives   0101001010001000010001100

INCENTIVE	EFFECTIVENESS
1. Vendor penalty for late implementation	**PRO:** Encourages the vendor to prioritize your delivery and installation if behind schedule. **CON:** May lead to finger pointing; involves constant documentation of things the vendor fails to do that may cause a delay.
2. Mutual bonus and penalty opportunity	**PRO:** Encourages everyone to support the same goal. **CON:** May be difficult to construct; provider leadership may not be willing to pay a penalty to the vendor for the provider's failure to perform.

Reprinted with permission, Boundary Information Group

approach lines up the incentives for both the provider and vendor to work together to achieve the bonus. The provider sets aside a portion of money that could be paid out as a bonus to both the vendor and the provider (often the provider project implementation team). The format of this incentive program is shown in Exhibit 6.13.

EXHIBIT 6.13   Mutual Incentive Format   1001010010000100011001

	VENDOR DOES NOT MEET GOALS	VENDOR MEETS/EXCEEDS GOALS
PROVIDER DOES NOT MEET GOALS	No incentive payments	Incentive paid to vendor
PROVIDER MEETS/EXCEEDS GOALS	Vendor pays incentive to provider	Incentive paid to vendor and provider

Reprinted with permission, Boundary Information Group

The bottom line of the negotiations is to form a relationship that leads to the provider achieving its goals and the vendor achieving its business objectives (including making a profit and having a satisfied customer). If the negotiations are not headed in that direction, pause to see whether there is a way to address or neutralize the issues that appear to be important to one party and a problem for the other. During the negotiations, limit discussions of the details to only those who need to know. Both parties will be best served by being able to accept and endorse the final agreement once the negotiated agreement is approved by the top executives or board and an authorized officer of the vendor. Then you have an agreement that forms the basis for moving forward to implementation.

▶ Conclusion

Technology planning, selection, and negotiations are complex processes. They are even more complex for EHRs in this decade because, for most providers, the products selected are the first robust EHR applications in their environment. Thus, the EHR implementation process includes creating and maintaining a solid technical infrastructure to support the EHR, including modification of existing paper-based work flows and data flows to transition into an environment that supports electronic data and work flow management. Selecting the right vendor, product mix, and infrastructure are important key elements to the successful transformation of your practice into an environment that effectively utilizes an EHR. The next chapter, which discusses the implementation process, is another important step in this transformation.

NOTES

1. Amatayakul, M, *Electronic Health Records: A Practical Guide for Professionals and Organizations*, Second Edition, Chicago: American Health Information Management Association, 2004, pp 229-251; Baum, N, "EMR: A Big Investment with an Excellent Return," *Private Practice Success*, April 2003, pp 8-9; Holly, J, "Through the Barrier of Financial Constraints," *Advance for Health Information Executives*, May 2003, pp 26, 28, 30.

2. Go to the HL7 Electronic Health Record Web page (www.hl7.org/EHR) and select Downloads.

3. Jewson Enterprises (www.jewsonenterprises.com).

4. KLAS Enterprises, LLC (www.healthcomputing.com/site/v2).

5. Chin, T, "Financing High-Tech: You Can Afford It After All." Available at www.ama-assn.org/amednews/2004/03/08/bisa0308.htm, 47(10).

6. "How Are You Going to Pay for That EMR System?" *Advisory Publications*, September 2002, pp 4-5.

7. Daigrepont, J, "EMR Pitfalls: Avoiding Costly Purchasing Mistakes," *Journal of Medical Practice Management*, September/October 2003, 19(2), pp 80-83.

8. Valancy, J, "How Much Will That EMR System Really Cost?" *Family Practice Management*, April 2002, pp 57-58.

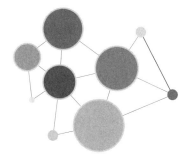

▶ SEVEN

Planning and Initiating an EHR Implementation

This chapter discusses EHR implementation through final testing, at which point you should be prepared to go live with the EHR. Most group practices implementing EHRs will be converting clinical data from paper records. If you are also implementing a practice management system (PMS) before or at the same time as the EHR, however, most of the same steps will apply. The data conversion preparation may be different in that you are likely to be converting some of your PMS data electronically from the current system.

THIS CHAPTER HELPS you in planning and initiating your EHR implementation by presenting methods to:

- ▶ Use a structured project plan;
- ▶ Assign staff and allocate resources;
- ▶ Determine your responsibilities and what to expect from your vendor in terms of installation, testing, updates, and responsibility;
- ▶ Plan and monitor a budget for EHR implementation;
- ▶ Deal with technical issues;
- ▶ Determine work flow with the EHR and customization according to your practice's needs and desires;
- ▶ Plan for installation, testing, and training; and
- ▶ Convert data from paper and other formats to the EHR.

▶ The EHR Project Plan

The EHR project plan should provide a common reference point for the following types of information:

- ▶ The timing of each major task, milestone, and deliverable;

- ▶ Identification of the person with the lead responsibility for organizing and completing each task;

- ▶ The beginning and end dates of each task;

- ▶ The dependency relationship of the beginning of one task based on the completion of one or more (precedent) tasks; and

- ▶ An accounting of the status of each task in the project at any specific time.

It is important to use a structured project plan. The vendor, your group practice, and other support and services involved in the EHR implementation will need to schedule resources and allocate them to the project. Consider using project management software with access afforded to all of the key individuals involved.

A sample of the project plan sections for an EHR is shown in Exhibit 7.1.

The project plan may include additional information about resources allocated to the task. The overall project information provides the project manager with the basis not only to manage the project but also to communicate effectively with all other team leaders and key participants regarding schedule and resource issues. The project management team should note and handle any variance from the project plan to keep the project on schedule.

Another key component of project management involves the budget and expenditures. Just as the time and staffing resources associated with any large project task should be managed, in a project as complex as an EHR implementation, the budget and expenditures should be tracked on at least a monthly basis. The project management team, perhaps together with the chief financial officer (CFO), should manage any variation from the expected expenses.

EXHIBIT 7.1   EHR Project Plan Sample Content   001000010001100

MAJOR PROJECT PLAN SECTIONS:

- ▶ Periodic project management and team meetings
- ▶ Infrastructure
  - ▷ Wired
  - ▷ Wireless
  - ▷ Network upgrades and testing
- ▶ Hardware – delivery, installation, and testing
  - ▷ Servers
  - ▷ End-user devices
  - ▷ Other hardware, including printers
- ▶ Work flow – analysis, design, and build
- ▶ Data flow – analysis, design, and build
- ▶ Data dictionary – design and build
- ▶ Data warehouse – design and build
- ▶ HIPAA Security and Privacy Rules policies and procedures – review and modification
- ▶ Testing – design and build
- ▶ Pilot(s) – design and build
- ▶ Data conversion – plan and test
- ▶ Training – design, build, and test
- ▶ Interfaces – design, build, and test

Reprinted with permission, Boundary Information Group

▶ Allocation of Internal Staff and External Resources

Most organizations implementing an EHR use a combination of internal staff and external resources. To the greatest extent possible, use internal resources for the decisions regarding work flow and data conversion, the support of hardware and software upgrades, and end-user training. These areas are specific to the culture of the organization as well as the ongoing technical and end-user support for the EHR.

To keep the implementation on schedule, be sure you have adequate personnel resources. In addition, a mix of knowledge and capabilities are key to identifying the implications of the options available during implementation and recommending strategies that are best for the organization.

Exhibit 7.2 presents a sample list of personnel resources. Use this list as a starting point to identify the personnel that you and the vendor will use on this project.

A designated project manager should lead the project management team. If the team approach is used, allocate at least one person full-time to manage the project. In larger organizations, a multi-person full-time project team approach is often used, with clinical personnel participating on the team. Note that such complex information systems (IS) projects as EHRs often go astray or take much longer than expected because the personnel assigned

EXHIBIT 7.2   Sample Checklist for Personnel Resources 10001100

PERSONNEL RESOURCE	% TIME	NAME
STAFF		
❏ EHR project manager		
❏ Health information management / Medical records		
❏ Clinical operations		
❏ Clinician(s)		
❏ IT network		
❏ IT database		
❏ IT end-user support		
❏ Trainer		
❏ Other		
VENDOR		
❏ EHR project manager		
❏ Technical installation		
❏ User/Application installation		
❏ Trainer		
❏ Interface programmer		
❏ Other		
OTHER		
❏ IT consultant		
❏ EHR applications consultant		

Reprinted with permission, Boundary Information Group

to the project are not allocated full-time, or they are not relieved of enough other duties and responsibilities to spend the time planned on this project.

External resources can be extremely helpful on an interim basis during the implementation project to provide the following:

▶ Additional labor hours when internal personnel are not sufficiently available to the project;

▶ Expertise from previous EHR and similar installations;

▶ Solid project management and budget management skills; and

▶ Problem resolution management, especially with issues on which the vendor and practice do not agree, or if there is a lack of consensus within the practice on how to proceed.

One way to determine the size and level of effort expected from the project team is to solicit information from the references provided by the EHR vendor as well as the organizations where site visits were conducted. Do not be surprised if others tell you that they tried to make do with a smaller implementation team, found that it was not working, and had to increase the level of effort. (It is common for physician practices and hospitals to try to cut back the amount of staff time allocated or the consultant/vendor time contracted, with the expectation of saving money, and then to find that the staff that have been allocated aren't sufficient to keep the project on schedule.) Your practice has the responsibility to make its allocated staff available on a continuing basis to support the project at a level commensurate with the work required.

You can take two steps to help ensure that the vendor provides experienced personnel for leadership positions. First, include in your RFP a requirement that the team leaders be experienced and that you have the right to reasonably request the vendor to replace any assigned personnel who, in your opinion, are either not qualified to do the work assigned or are not working well with your staff. Establish in your RFP the experience qualifications of the key vendor personnel who will participate in your implementation, including the vendor project manager, implementation team leaders, technical support leaders and training leaders. It is unreasonable, however, to expect resumes of specific individuals to be included in the vendor's proposal because usually four to six months go by between the time the proposals are submitted and work starts on the implementation. The vendor staff assigned to your project therefore will be partially determined by which staff are available when the work begins.

Second, you can require (during or immediately after contract negotiations) that you have an opportunity to review the resumes of the vendor's proposed team leaders and have the right to interview these people by telephone. The proposed personnel should have actual experience with the vendor's product in the areas where they are assigned, as well as overall work experience. It is also appropriate to ask for a limited number of references. Remember, however, that you are not interviewing these individuals to accept a permanent position in your organization. The vendor has significant responsibility to assure that individuals assigned are available, productive, and qualified. The practice's primary concern with these personnel should be their experience with the vendor product and the amount of training they have had on the product.

▶ Expectations from Your Vendor

Your vendor supports many customers, and probably is constantly in the process of improving its software products with updates and new versions. Vendors are not perfect, but a large number of them have products that work reasonably well, and they have the on-site and off-site personnel to resolve their product problems as well as help in addressing internal problems that will arise during the implementation. Interfaces to other vendor products that you already use, such as a PMS, may also present issues. In some cases your EHR vendor will have a successful track record with these other products; in other cases, the vendor will not. Unless you contract for your EHR vendor to directly develop, manage, and test the interfaces to the other vendor products, you have the primary responsibility for ensuring that all of your vendors can and will work together to achieve a successful implementation.

Exhibit 7.3 presents a sample list of expectations of your EHR vendor. Remember, though, the vendor also has expectations of you. Very often, in the vendor's proposal or EHR implementation manual, the major responsibilities of your practice as well as those of the vendor will be spelled out. In some cases the areas of responsibility will be defined as being joint efforts. The clearer that these responsibilities are specified in writing and well understood prior to the implementation, the better the implementation will go for both parties.

Your RFP expresses your requirements, and the vendor's response describes how it will address each of your requirements. Most of the time, through RFP responses, vendor demonstrations, and site visits, an organization can

EXHIBIT 7.3 Example Expectations of Your EHR Vendor 00011001

> ▶ On-time delivery and installation of hardware that functions per the contracted terms;
>
> ▶ On-time delivery and installation of software that functions per the contracted terms;
>
> ▶ An implementation project plan customized to your practice;
>
> ▶ Support for data conversion, work flow analysis, and EHR setup to support your practice's vision;
>
> ▶ Help with interfaces to your PMS, diagnostic equipment, and external trading partners (e.g., lab, pharmacy);
>
> ▶ Resolution of vendor product problems in a reasonable amount of time;
>
> ▶ Support to help you identify and resolve your practice's internal implementation problems and those of third parties (e.g., interfaces to your PMS vendor); and
>
> ▶ Adherence to data and transaction standards required per your RFP.

Reprinted with permission, Boundary Information Group

obtain a realistic picture of the vendor's software capability, hardware requirements, and performance metrics (e.g., response time). If, during this process, you can identify deficiencies the vendor has agreed to address (e.g., the vendor's current version does not meet your full requirements for a function in the EHR software that is important to you, but they agree to resolve the issue within six months or a year), then you can expect the vendor's implementation plan to include responses to such issues. You can also negotiate to withhold some money due the vendor until an issue is resolved to your satisfaction.

Two other areas of vendor expectations are often more difficult to address. The first deals with the project plan. Your vendor's proposal should include a model project plan that specifies the responsibilities and time frames for tasks for both the vendor and the practice. To achieve a successful EHR implementation, both the vendor and your organization need to provide the necessary resources to execute the project plan together. Second, you should monitor the vendor's ability to supply the qualified personnel according to the schedule of the plan. It is helpful to have continuity of vendor personnel working on your implementation project to the extent that the individuals are qualified to work on multiple components. The contract should clearly state the expected work schedule of the vendor personnel, including the degree to which they will be working on site vs. off site. If personnel work off site, their billable hours should be documented to your satisfaction, and the contract should also clearly state this requirement.

▶ Planning and Monitoring the Budget

Chapter 6, How to Select the Right Vendor and EHR for Your Practice, describes the construction of the budget for implementation and ongoing operations. A significant part of the budget addresses payments that you make to the vendor, but these are not the only budget components. You should set up a monitoring program to track actual expenses against budget. Depending on the size of your organization and its sensitivity to monitoring the EHR project, you should expect to update and monitor actual expenses vs. budget on a monthly basis and to report the status to the CFO or administrator and others on a monthly or quarterly basis. You may want to consider tracking the expense vs. budget in two ways. The traditional method of tracking budget vs. expense by time, usually on a monthly basis, works well if everything on the project remains on schedule. However, some slippage is not unusual, which might provide a false sense of expenses being within budget, based on time, when expenses are actually over budget when compared to project progress to date. Therefore, you should also have a second budget management report, which compares budget to actual expenses based on progress to date.

If you have an incentive-based project, or you have withholds in your EHR contract, do not forget to include the incentive and withhold payments due based on deliverables to date, even though you have not yet paid out the money. You may need to set up a spreadsheet to track the progress-based budget vs. expense budget for the EHR project to take all of these factors into consideration. Your vendor may have templates that can be helpful. If the project management team is not skilled in designing templates to achieve these monitoring objectives, your CFO or administrator may be able to help in setting up the methodology.

Exhibit 7.4 illustrates the importance of monitoring EHR expenditures against budget by both time and progress. The upper two sections of the exhibit display the cumulative budget per quarter, as well as the actual expenses per quarter and the actual cumulative expenses. Six months into the project, actual expenses are $245,000, which compares favorably with a time-based budget of $250,000. The lower half of the exhibit displays the budgeted expenses based on progress. This budget cannot be prepared until the progress is known at the end of each quarter. It shows the budget based on progress cumulative through the first six months to be $210,000. The last section of the exhibit indicates that, based on progress, the project is in a $35,000 overrun situation. In complex projects such as an EHR, where all of the activities are not likely to occur on schedule, this budget analysis against progress is an important tool to monitor not only major milestones that are behind schedule, but to understand the financial impacts to date based on work completed.

EXHIBIT 7.4   Budget Monitoring Example: 001010010000100011001
EHR Budget by Quarter

	QUARTER 1	QUARTER 2	QUARTER 3	QUARTER 4
EHR Budget/Quarter	$100,000	$150,000	$150,000	$200,000
EHR Budget Cumulative	$100,000	$250,000	$400,000	$600,000
Actual Expenses/Quarter	$85,000	$160,000		
Actual Expenses Cumulative	$85,000	$245,000		
EHR Progress Budget/Quarterly	$90,000	$120,000		
EHR Progress Budget Cumulative	$90,000	$210,000		
Variance Progress Expenses vs. Budget	$5,000	($40,000)		
Variance Cumulative Progress vs. Budget	$5,000	$35,000		

Reprinted with permission, Boundary Information Group

► Technical Issues for Consideration

A number of key technical issues are important in supporting the EHR. Many of them will apply to your EHR implementation.

- ► *Wireless technology*, including security and speed, is particularly useful for mobile notepads and tablets (real-time wireless or batch wireless, with sufficient screen size to be read and used by physicians and other clinicians).

- ► *Network capacity management* includes monitoring the network bandwidth and assessing the need to increase capacity based on the volume of traffic and size of message packets (e.g., scanned electronic image documents are much bigger than digital documents).

▶ *Remote access* to the EHR (by clinicians, IS staff, and perhaps others) implies the need for a security review and perhaps the use of additional precautions. Organizations commonly use two-tiered secured user access. The two tiers are usually something the user knows and something the user has.[1] For example, the user commonly knows a password, and the characteristic that the user has can be a security token that changes keys every minute or so. It can also be a biometric (e.g., a fingerprint), although the use of biometrics is not widespread at this time. Also consider a configuration review of the firewall or an upgrade to the firewall, based on the scope of use by remote access. Note that remote access could also occur if you operate clinics in remote facilities, such as a school or a senior center. In this case, one option to consider is to access the EHR through the same mechanisms used by staff for remote access from home.

Key Technical Issues
▶ Wireless technology
▶ Network capacity
▶ Access
▶ Thick vs. thin clients
▶ Network bandwidth
▶ Storage configuration

▶ *Thick clients* are traditional desktop PCs or laptops in which the machine stores all of its operating system software and all of its applications, and can even store the data on a hard drive. Often, thick clients store data on a server either during or after processing is completed, but they basically are full stand-alone systems.

▶ *Thin clients* are bare bones laptops and desktop computers that have a processor and very little storage ability. Thin clients depend on the servers in the network to perform their processing functions and store data. Thin clients are generally lower in cost than thick clients because they don't have all the functionality of the thick client. Thin clients are also generally considered more secure because they do not permit downloading of data onto portable storage media or transmission of data except through the central servers. This reduces the likelihood that someone could steal data, and it greatly reduces the potential for the introduction of viruses via portable storage media. Although some EHR application software is designed to work well on thin clients, that is not true for all EHR software. Some thin-client users also find a small amount of lag time in processing data because there is no local processing capability.

It is possible to mix the use of thick and thin clients on the same network. For instance, staff in financial services or the business office may require workstation-supported applications that are not shared with others (thick clients), whereas the clinicians and registration personnel might utilize thin client devices. Two important questions to consider when choosing thick vs. thin client uses for an EHR and PMS are: Will the vendor application software support one or both options? Is there a significant difference to the clinicians in response time with the use of thick vs. thin clients for the clinical applications that they use? Note that applications other than the PMS and EHR could drive the choice of device client.

▶ The *network bandwidth* should be analyzed based on the amount of traffic on the network and the type of traffic. For instance, an EHR based almost entirely on digital data will not require the same network capacity as an EHR based significantly on scanned documents. Consideration regarding scanned documents needs to include the paper document conversion plan on implementation and the ongoing reliance of scanned vs. digital data. For example, if laboratory reports are received in paper form and scanned into the EHR, then most charts will have a lot of scanned documents with laboratory data, which may be accessed frequently. In contrast, laboratory data supplied digitally directly from the major laboratories or paper reports keyed directly into the EHR laboratory result form or template used for the electronic patient chart result in less capacity demand on the network. The use of thick vs. thin clients has an impact on the network bandwidth requirements. Network technicians can help analyze the need to base the network on a T1, T3, fiber-optic, or other technology. The experience of other comparable-sized organizations using a similar EHR document strategy could provide considerable insight.

▶ The recommended *technical storage configuration* for active records in the EHR is dual processors or a cluster of servers. The EHR must be operational for patient records to be accessible, so moderate or lengthy downtimes pose significant problems for the organization because clinicians will not have access to patient data. It is therefore important to minimize the probability of downtime during working hours and to minimize the amount of time to restore access to patient data, taking into account cost. A common approach to address these issues is to use dual processors that simultaneously record all data in a clinical data repository (CDR) and are configured with an automatic switchover from one processor to the other in the case of failure. Evaluate the configuration of servers, along with the capabilities of the EHR to best support reporting and the business needs of the organization.[2] Consider including a separate clinical and financial data warehouse server for financial and clinical reporting.

These foregoing examples of technology considerations that your practice will face while implementing the EHR require the services of knowledgeable personnel. You may need to hire additional staff with technical capabilities in one or more of these areas, seek assistance from your EHR vendor, and/or obtain help from technology consultants in your community. Many of the technologies described here are different from those that you have been using for your PMS because the work flow of the clinicians is different from that of your administrative staff in a number of ways. For example:

▶ The clinicians are mobile whereas most of the administrative staff are stationary (mobile wireless vs. desktop);

▶ Clinicians may prefer point-and-click entry and retrieval to support digital data, and they may prefer a smaller device without a keyboard;

▶ Clinicians may be using images and/or scanned documents to a greater extent than the administrative staff, requiring increased bandwidth;

▶ Server redundancy is more important for clinical applications because the consequences of downtime are more significant; or

▶ Adding physicians and other clinicians to the infrastructure increases the number of users significantly, which may contribute to the need for additional support personnel and increased network capacity.

Undoubtedly, through the increased use of the Internet, wireless devices, and other technologies, you will need to periodically review technology considerations based on changes in options and costs. Initially in the implementation, you should give high priority to technologies that are well established in comparable organizations for purposes similar to yours. A substantial number of EHR project implementation risks are inherent in the cultural changes, people involved, and technologies without further complicating the implementation with unproven technology (unless it is inevitable because there is no proven technology for a required business purpose).

▶ Changes in Job Descriptions and Policies and Procedures for the EHR

Most organizations find that some job descriptions change with the use of an EHR; in some cases, job descriptions must be created for positions that did not exist before. For instance, most medium to large-size organizations with an EHR have one or more database administrators (DBAs) and/or health data analysts (HDAs). In part, personnel in these positions may perform some of the duties that were previously performed by individuals dedicated to writing reports. The relational database EHR should provide the tools and infrastructure support so that your management staff and clinicians can generate their own standard reports. In addition, the ability to conduct special reports quickly is significant.

As an example, a 50-physician cardiology practice had implemented an EHR for about a year when a relatively new drug used in treating cardiology patients was recalled. The day the recall was issued, all of the electronic patient records were searched to identify the patients who had been prescribed that drug. In less than an hour, a list was prepared of all of the patients who did not have an appointment scheduled in the following week. That same day, all of these patients were called and scheduled to see their physicians within a few days. This report certainly had not been planned as part of the EHR implementation. But because the practice had its own DBA, utilized a point-and-click system that specifically identified each drug and dosage prescribed, and used a relational database, it was able to provide better patient care than if it had not had an EHR. Searching through the old paper record system would have been cost prohibitive. Other cardiology practices without an EHR would have just waited until the patients showed up for their next visits to review medications, and if necessary changed the drug then.

DBAs are used in all industries. An HDA position is similar but has more emphasis on understanding the construction and use of health care data and less direct expertise in the technical aspects of relational databases. Exhibit 7.5 on pages 188–89 shows a sample job description for an HDA.

EXHIBIT 7.5   Sample Job Description for a Health Data Analyst 10100

JOB TITLE: Health Data Analyst

GENERAL SUMMARY OF DUTIES: Responsible for planning, organizing, and monitoring the data dictionary, database(s), and report management for the organization's business and clinical data.

SUPERVISION RECEIVED: Reports to the _____

SUPERVISION EXERCISED: Serves as a team leader on occasion

ESSENTIAL FUNCTIONS:
1. Manages the electronic databases for the PMS, EHR, clinical data repository, and other enterprise databases.
2. May manage department specific databases.
3. Maintains the data dictionary for the enterprise and each application.
4. Monitors regulatory and standards changes that impact data definitions used internally and in the exchange of data with external organizations.
5. Maintains database integrity.
6. Designs and maintains management reports for clinical and administrative staff.
7. Supports staff in the design of data collection, storage, and use.
8. Meets with users to gather reporting requirements, analyzes the requirements, and formulates a plan to develop the data and report procedures to satisfy the requirements.
9. Provides basic training on report writing and use for new report users, ensuring that all users are aware of and trained on the use of reports.

The job holder must demonstrate competencies applicable to the job description.

EDUCATION: Associate or bachelor's degree in health administration, business administration, statistics, informatics, or related field. Professional development courses in health data management desirable.

EXPERIENCE: Minimum of two years health care data analysis experience in a physician practice or hospital.

REQUIREMENTS: None

KNOWLEDGE:
1. Familiarity with HIPAA (transactions and) code sets standards, and procedure, diagnosis and billing code sets, preferred.
2. Knowledge of computer systems, programs, databases, and report writing.
3. Knowledge of the principles of data integrity.

continued next page

EXHIBIT 7.5   Sample Job Description for a Health Data Analyst *cont.*

4. Knowledge of minicomputer and personal computer environments, architecture, and functions.
5. Knowledge of report writing software.

SKILLS:
1. Skill in establishing and maintaining effective working relationships.
2. Skill in organizing work and achieving goals and objectives.
3. Skill in paying attention to detail, including finding and correcting data errors and reporting programming errors.
4. Skill in dealing with application capabilities required in database, spreadsheet, and word processing.
5. Skill in using customer service techniques.

ABILITIES:
1. Ability to organize and prioritize projects and assignments.
2. Ability to utilize statistics principles in preparing data and reports.
3. Ability to maintain strict confidentiality with patient and clinic data.
4. Ability to exercise professionalism when interacting with physicians, staff, and external customers.
5. Ability to explain data analysis topics clearly and simply, verbally, and in writing.

ENVIRONMENTAL/WORKING CONDITIONS: Office setting

PHYSICAL/MENTAL DEMANDS: Sitting for prolonged periods at a computer terminal, stooping, bending, and twisting. Requires ability to lift or push up to 20 pounds. Occasional stress in dealing with multiple tasks.

This description is intended to provide only basic guidelines for meeting job requirements. Responsibilities, knowledge, skills, abilities, and working conditions may change as needs evolve.

Reprinted with permission, Boundary Information Group

The job descriptions of some of the medical record staff are likely to be changed. For instance, they may become the data entry personnel for clinical information received on paper from external sources (e.g., paper lab results). They are often the individuals designated to separate the data from two patients that have been placed in one EHR patient record or to merge together two EHR patient records on the same patient. They have performed this same function for paper charts, and these problems will continue to occur, although perhaps on a less frequent basis. Multiple charts are often created for the same patient with paper chart systems because the known paper chart cannot be found so a second one is created; this problem is reduced significantly with the EHR (see the section "Tools for Managing EHRs" later in this chapter).

Positions in the organization that are likely to be reduced in number or eliminated include transcriptionists and the couriers who move charts from one location to another in a multi-location practice. EHRs usually require additional technical and electronic data management support and perhaps additional training capability.

All of your policies and procedures, including those for HIPAA Privacy and Security Rules, should be reviewed to reflect the administrative, work flow, and technical changes that you implement with your EHR. For instance, in a paper-based medical record practice, you may have different sanctions and a different reporting process for individuals who look at patient charts for which they have no treatment or other business relationship. Because paper charts often are tightly controlled by medical record staff, your policies may be more directed toward how the medical records staff allow access to the charts than to the individual responsibilities of your workforce. In an EHR environment, all members of your workforce potentially have access to the system, so technical controls must be in place, but due to the usual implementation of an emergency "break the glass" capability, all physicians and sometimes other clinicians often have access to records for patients they are not treating or for whom they do not have another business need. These accesses also need to be controlled and monitored. Most practices and hospitals implement a combination of audit trails and automatic reporting of these instances so they can be monitored by a responsible individual, who is not necessarily part of the medical records team.[3]

▶ Installing and Testing Equipment and Software

Your implementation should not proceed without successfully testing every component combination in your testing plan. Your EHR vendor should have a plan for delivering and testing the vendor's equipment and software. You may have to work with the vendor to develop a plan to test your existing network, workstations, and interfaces to products from other vendors to make sure that they work properly in conjunction the EHR application and have the capacity to handle the increased volume of data communication.

You and your vendor should have an approved testing plan. These plans often include the use of test data for which the expected results of the tests are known to make sure they can be duplicated. You can use real data for some components of the system to test whether they produce the same results as your legacy systems using the same data.

A "load" test may require several staff members spending a number of hours entering and accessing data simultaneously to replicate the volume of data that you expect in your practice post-EHR implementation. This type of load testing is particularly helpful for assessing the network capacity, as well as the wireless communications and server data communications capacity.

▶ Assigning Responsibility for Installation

Responsibility for the installation of the EHR, from ordering the components to being ready to go live, is a joint responsibility of the vendor and the practice. Even if the practice has outsourced a significant part of the support for the implementation to the vendor, the two organizations still share responsibility for the implementation. That means that your clinicians and administrative staff have to be involved in key aspects of the process to get all of the

001010010110100101001010010100100

Involve Your Staff

Vendors cannot successfully implement systems in the absence of active customer participation. The EHR will work only if your users have participated in designing and testing the EHR.

systems, work flow, and training completed before implementation. Most organizations significantly share in the responsibility for the installation because the practice will have the major responsibility for maintaining the system after implementation has been completed. To best learn and understand how the EHR works, how it fits together with other systems and hardware, and what the work flow will be to meet the business objectives of your practice, your staff should be actively engaged in the design and decision-making processes that occur during the implementation phase.

▶ Creating Decision Rules and Work Flow Templates for Your Practice

Most EHR vendors have specialty-specific templates that can be used as starting points for creating the work flow pattern, which varies by specialty to some degree. For instance, primary care and some specialty practices, such as cardiology, have a lot of activity associated with prescription refills by telephone. Often, one or more nurses assigned to the prescription refill activity can access the records electronically while the pharmacy or patient is on the phone, which improves the work flow process significantly. This aspect might be of little interest, however, to surgeons, who usually don't have patients calling in for prescription refills. Exhibit 7.6 shows a sample checklist of work flow improvement opportunities.

EXHIBIT 7.6   Common Work Flow Improvement Opportunities

WORK FLOW OPPORTUNITIES	OUR PRACTICE (Y/N)
1. Physician in-box messages	
2. Processing prescription refill requests	
3. Lab results management	
4. Physician orders to nurses, technicians, etc.	
5. Retrieval of patient chart for office visit	
6. Follow-up visit documentation and comparison of previous data	
7. Recording vital signs and problem list and communicating to the physician	
8. Disease management of patients with chronic conditions	

Reprinted with Permission, Boundary Information Group

Your clinicians must make a number of decisions with regard to how data will be recorded and presented. These decisions will go into the templates you use, which will be unique to your practice. It is recommended, however, that the templates not be customized to individual physicians because this can present training, help desk, and other significant support issues for your practice to address at additional cost.

It is important for patient safety and beneficial for your practice to define each of the data elements the same, no matter where they are used. It is best if the group practice leadership approves, as one of the goals of the EHR, the use of standard data throughout the organization. It then becomes a top-down approach for your EHR implementation. With a data standardization objective, one of the responsibilities of the practice implementation team is to create a structure and process to resolve non-standard use of terminology so the organization can proceed with a single set of data dictionary terms and definitions. In some cases, this will help reduce the fraud and abuse potential regarding billing because there will be a enterprise-wide definition of terms as they are used for recording procedures, diagnoses, and other documentation for billing purposes.

▶ Pilot Testing the EHR in Your Practice

Another important part of project management is testing the EHR before going "live." Together with the vendor, you should develop a pilot testing plan to make sure that all of the functionality of the EHR is working before going into production. Testing should include the following concerns (as examples):

- ▶ Do the data entry devices work in each setting?

- ▶ Can data be entered and retrieved correctly?

- ▶ Do data pass correctly from the EHR to the PMS for billing purposes?

- ▶ Can the PMS correctly create an 837P electronic claims transaction and either receive or send the other HIPAA transactions your practice has chosen to implement?

- ▶ Can demographic, clinical, and financial data that are entered be retrieved through a third-party report management tool into report formats that are populated correctly with the test data?

- ▶ Do the PMS and EHR response times meet your standards?

- ▶ Can each specialty physician in your practice document history, physical, diagnosis, and treatment in a data sequence and work flow that is productive?

- ▶ Can the clinicians in each specialty in your practice retrieve data on specific patients quickly and easily?

► Can clinicians in each specialty in your practice retrieve their messages, results to be reviewed, and other electronic incoming messages in a work flow that is productive for them without losing any messages?

As an option, consider surveying the patients who are treated during the pilot to see if they have any positive or negative feelings associated with being involved in clinical encounters in a practice in which a computing device is used.

► Planning for Training

Training is an important resource for a successful EHR implementation as well as for ongoing maintenance. At least one trainer should be designated for the EHR implementation, with additional individuals serving as backups. The EHR trainer should be a clinician because physicians, dentists, and other clinicians will feel most comfortable being trained by a clinician. In addition, a clinician will be familiar with how to best implement the work flow tools and patient records data into a clinician's functions. To the greatest extent possible, the customization of the implementation should be kept simple, with the flow of screens as well as retrieval and storage of data being as intuitive as possible.

Your key in-house trainers will first require training from the vendor. (This may be provided at your site or in a vendor-specified location.) In addition, members of the implementation team and EHR project team may benefit from education and training on the use and operation of EHRs, either from your vendor, from professional associations, or from other sources. The EHR budget should provide funds for registration fees and travel for appropriate training in this regard, as well as the purchase of books and participation in audio-conferences and other learning experiences that will help the staff understand how to best approach this project.

► EHR Implementation and Paper Chart Conversion

Converting the Paper Charts

One of the most important decisions in implementing an EHR is to decide how to convert the paper charts. At least three different approaches exist for converting the paper chart data. Some have different options, as seen in the following list:

1. *Scanning.* The method of scanning the paper chart is easy to do and involves no downtime for physicians and other clinicians in terms of moving the data from the paper chart to the EHR. If this strategy is used, consider employing a scanning service from the EHR vendor or third party to temporarily provide high-speed scanners and staff to scan the documents into the EHR. The documents must be indexed as part of the scanning process so they can be retrieved later. Of course, the more customization of the index, beyond identifying the patient, date, and type of document, the greater the setup time and labor involved in the process. For help in determining how to best index the documents, consult users who have implemented the same EHR and have taken a scanning approach, or ask the vendor.

    A second option for accomplishing scanning is to scan the patient paper charts the day before patients are scheduled for their first appointments after the conversion. This spreads out the scanning process and workload, but it also lengthens the time to complete the process. In the first option, once all of the records are scanned, they are accessible anytime and anywhere by any authorized user. With the second option, it can be a year or longer before all of the records are available electronically, and until that time the practice is using a less desirable dual system (see the section "Operating Dual Systems during the Transition" at the end of this chapter).

2. *Abstracting.* A second approach is to create an abstract of information from the paper chart that is digitally completed in the EHR. A sample checklist for an abstract is shown in Exhibit 7.7 on the next page.

3. *Combination of selective scanning and abstracting.* A third approach is to use an abstract together with scanning selected documents. This approach has two options. One option is for the physicians to specify criteria to be used by the medical records staff to create the abstract data and select the documents from the paper chart that are to be scanned into the EHR. This should be tested as part of a pilot implementation of the EHR before deploying it enterprise-wide. To some extent, the success or failure of this approach depends on the quality and specificity of the guidelines developed by the physicians and the clinical knowledge of the medical records staff.

    A second option is to schedule physicians for one-half to three-quarters of a patient load for the first two weeks of implementation

EXHIBIT 7.7 EHR Abstract Checklist Sample `1010010000010001100`

1. Patient name
   ▶ First name
   ▶ Middle initial/Name
   ▶ Last name
2. Patient/Chart ID number (account number)
3. Date of birth
4. Gender
5. Address
   ▶ Street
   ▶ Apartment
   ▶ City
   ▶ State
   ▶ Zip Code
6. Parent/Guardian (if applicable)
   ▶ Name
   ▶ Relationship
7. Phone number
   ▶ Home
   ▶ Work
   ▶ Cell
8. Current medications (including over-the-counter)
   ▶ Name
   ▶ Dosage
   ▶ Frequency
   ▶ Last prescription date
9. Allergies
   ▶ Allergy
   ▶ Reaction
10. Height and date
11. Weight and date
12. Hair color (optional)
13. Eye color (optional)
14. Chronic diagnoses and problems
15. Last encounter
    ▶ Date
    ▶ Reason
16. Last Diagnostic/Procedures, date, and major findings
    ▶ Complete H & P (patient history and physical examination)
    ▶ Mammography
    ▶ PAP (papanicolaou) test
    ▶ PSA (prostate-specific antigen) test
    ▶ Colonoscopy/Sigmoidoscopy
17. Immunizations

Reprinted with permission, Boundary Information Group

(which could be staggered by location). This provides the physicians with extra time between patients to allow for an initial (slower than normal) process of documentation and getting used to the system. For new patients, physicians can normally document right in the EHR. For all follow-up patients, the staff provide the physician the paper chart together with a brief abstract. While treating the patient, the physician can note which documents within the paper chart should be scanned for the EHR and add to the abstract that has been prepared by the staff, if appropriate. This approach has temporary revenue loss implications, which should be included in the budget and return-on-investment (ROI) analysis.

Clinicians and medical records staff should collaborate on deciding which of these approaches will work best for the practice. If appropriate, a pilot for one or two of the approaches should be considered. The goal should be to find a paper chart conversion strategy, within a reasonable cost, that works well to preserve the patient documentation history but also allows for quickly finding the information in the EHR that clinicians need. The paper charts should be preserved for an appropriate period of time for backup and to meet any legal requirements for chart maintenance if the entire chart is not scanned. Depending on state and federal requirements, microfilming or scanned storage may be an option to off-site paper record storage.

Preloading Clinical Data

Another consideration for managing the EHR setup and ongoing use includes that of preloading some clinical data. Some providers find it advantageous to start populating the EHR with data before the conversion. For instance, electronic lab results from key outside labs could be implemented before conversion as long as there is a method for matching the patient's record number with the electronic results that are received. This may require some setup, which may not be practical until it occurs as part of the EHR implementation. It is a step to consider, however, if there would be value in having lab results preloaded in digital form before conversion for current use anytime, anywhere, as well as to provide additional electronic laboratory data for creating a longer history for clinical and quality of care study use.

▶ Testing the Data Conversion

No matter which method is used to convert data, the data conversion should be tested. If abstracting is used, a sample of abstracts should be validated against the original chart to make sure that the data are being abstracted completely and correctly. If document scanning is used, then a sample of the scanned documents (e.g., the documents for the first 200 patients) should be searched and retrieved from the EHR to be sure that all of the scanned documents actually entered the EHR and the documentation is complete on each patient. Establish a methodology to validate that the number of paper charts scanned match the number of EHR patient records with scanned documents.

A second step in testing the data conversion is to validate a sample of paper records against the EHR records to make sure the content in electronic form is readable (to the eye, in the case of scanned paper, handwritten and external documents; to the computer, in the case of digital documents such as abstracts or transcribed dictation). If the method used is the one for which old charts are scanned or abstracted the day before patients are seen for the first time after EHR implementation (instead of all at once during the implementation), there should be a mechanism to make sure that the number of paper charts scanned each day equals the number of new scanned charts in the EHR (adjusted for new patients seen for the first time, whose data are directly entered into the EHR).

▶ Tools for Managing EHRs

EHR tools for managing electronic records are another useful resource. In particular, just as in the paper chart world, it is possible for two electronic patient charts to be created for the same patient. This often happens in the paper world when a second chart is created because the practice can't find the first chart when the patient is seen. It can also happen when patient names are misspelled or patients don't correctly recall whether or when they have been seen before in the practice. When this happens in the paper chart world, and medical records verify that two charts are for the same person, the documentation in the charts is merged in paper form. The same process needs to happen in the EHR. Some EHR vendors provide tools to make this merging process easy once the match has been confirmed. There may be tools to search the EHR patient database to see if there are near characteristics of records in the repository that are candidates for a possible duplicate record (matching or closely matching names, date of birth, gender, telephone number, and so forth).

The other medical record problem that occurs in both the paper and electronic environments is that documents for different patients are filed in the same chart. In the paper chart world, the medical records staff go through the chart and separate the documents manually. In the electronic world, some EHR vendors provide tools to help facilitate that process. If your EHR vendor has such a tool, make sure that the appropriate staff know how to use it because it can be extremely helpful. These problems are usually identified by clinicians while they are treating patients, and they find something in the record that does not belong there. Or, such problems may be discovered through clinical data reporting, where edits are set to look for outliers and errors in the data. These incidents should happen less often in the electronic world than in the paper world. However, they still need to be managed because they occur in both environments.

▶ Testing and Implementing Interfaces

Most practices have a number of interfaces to implement in conjunction with the EHR. A sample of typical interfaces for medical practices is shown in Exhibit 7.8.

Some providers use an interface engine (a vendor-supplied product that manages and maintains the interfaces between applications within a hospital or group practice) to manage the internal process of moving data from

---

EXHIBIT 7.8   Examples of Interfaces to/from the EHR 010001100

- ▶ Practice management system
- ▶ E-prescribing to pharmacy
- ▶ External laboratory orders and reporting
- ▶ Internal laboratory orders and reporting
- ▶ Hospital(s)
- ▶ Data warehouse
- ▶ Radiology orders and reporting
- ▶ Health plan for eligibility, benefits, and preauthorization requirements

Reprinted with permission, Boundary Information Group

one application to another. Electronic interfaces to external trading partners are fairly new in the health care industry, except for the use of transactions between providers and health plans for billing, eligibility, and related purposes.

Some vendors offer a preprogrammed interface link between their application and the interface engine. These resources can be helpful in speeding up the interface implementation process and, to the extent the vendor maintains changes, can also assist with the maintenance function.

Each interface must be tested with the EHR before it can be implemented in a production mode. Physicians in some specialties may choose to implement electronic interfaces between their diagnostic equipment and the EHR. For instance, electrocardiogram (EKG) readings can be fed electronically from a machine appropriately equipped into the EHR. As you plan your EHR implementation, be sure to review the opportunities to use interfaces to improve work flow. You may decide to prioritize interface implementation based on cost, ease of implementation, and whether replacement equipment is required to accommodate the electronic data interface.

▶ Customizing the EHR to Support Your HIPAA Privacy and Security Policies and Procedures

The infrastructure of EHRs includes capabilities to support some aspects of the HIPAA Privacy and Security Rules. For instance, documentation by nurses and physicians needs to include a process for authenticating the individual, so the use of unique identifiers and passwords is inherent in the infrastructure. Most EHRs provide tools to identify individuals by roles, and manage work flow by role, thus supporting role-based access.

Because the EHR can provide new capabilities to administer HIPAA Privacy and Security Rules, you should review your current policies and procedures and your security risk analysis to see where the EHR can be customized to support your policies and procedures, as well as how it can be used to mitigate security risk. A typical example is the emergency access procedure, which is a required access control specification in the Security Rule. Many legacy systems do not provide for an emergency access procedure, but most EHRs do as this is a common business need. If your present HIPAA Privacy and Security policies and procedures have an administrative workaround for the emergency access procedure because you do not have a technical method for controlling the process, consider adopting a technical process based on the capability in your EHR and changing your HIPAA Privacy and Security policies and procedures to reflect this change.

▶ Operating Dual Systems during the Transition

Except for implementing EHRs in new organizations, the implementation process almost always involves operating dual systems over a short or long period of time. One of the systems is the EHR; the other is either a paper chart system, a documenting imaging system, an old EHR system that you are replacing, or a combination of partial EHR (e.g., electronic lab results) and paper charts. Usually, medical records staff are an important component of the team assembled to convert the data from paper to electronic form and to manage the dual system process.

A dual system can occur if a multi-site organization brings up the EHR one site at a time while some of the other sites are still operating on paper (especially when patients are seen at more than one site). A dual system also occurs when there is a deliberate strategy of converting paper charts to the EHR just before the first patient encounter after the implementation date, as discussed earlier. In this case, some patients have paper charts and others have electronic charts over a significant period of time. The dual systems approach is the only practical way for most group practices to convert to an EHR unless the conversion methodology is to scan all of the paper charts into an electronic format at one time.

Pay special attention to the following issues as long as any dual system process is in place:

▶ Convert the charts to the EHR and test them before they are needed by the clinician;

▶ Address non-encounter activities, such as telephone prescription refill requests from the patient, by a clear methodology so that staff know whether the chart is paper or in the EHR and whether this activity triggers a conversion from paper to electronic;

▶ Eliminate duplicate paper charts, to the greatest extent possible, prior to the conversion; and

▶ Specify an end point to the dual system operation at which time all remaining paper charts will be converted.

▶ Conclusion

Planning the implementation for an EHR is a multi-component process that requires a project management approach. One of the keys to success is involving a project management team representing key stakeholders in your organization. There are many important steps to a successful implementation. Good communication and collaboration between the practice and the vendor are essential. Studying work flow and designing improved work flow processes, as well as changing the organization's culture, take time, but they are essential to achieving the benefits of an EHR. Budget and progress management are important so that the EHR project remains on schedule, within budget, and focused on the established goals. Once the plan has been developed, the installation begun, and testing completed, you are ready to roll out the implementation.

NOTES

1. Amatayakul, M, SS Lazarus, T Walsh, and CP Hartley, *Handbook for HIPAA Security Implementation*, Chicago: AMA Press, 2004, p 115.

2. Amatayakul, M, *Electronic Health Records: A Practical Guide for Professionals and Organizations*, Second Edition, Chicago: American Health Information Management Association, 2004, pp 32-33.

3. Amatayakul, M, et al., *Handbook for HIPAA Security Implementation*, pp 143-144.

EIGHT

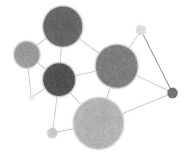

Implementation and Ongoing Operations – Going Live with Your EHR

Once all of the planning, preparation, and testing have been completed, you are ready to begin the production implementation of your EHR. This is a very sensitive and important aspect of EHR implementation because it can involve most, if not all, of your workforce. A significant allocation of resources from your organization and your vendor will have to be dedicated to this phase of the project due to the criticality of many of the initial steps of implementation. Once implementation is complete, resources are needed to keep the EHR running smoothly as well as to upgrade and expand its functionality.

THIS CHAPTER PROVIDES strategies for the EHR implementation phase and beyond. It helps you:

► Learn about the importance of converting data from the old system and testing the new system;

► Understand the need to have a phase-out of the old applications;

► Consider phasing in the implementation by location and/or department;

► Assess the value of building historical data prior to going live;

► Deploy training and support for the initial implementation, as well as staffing for EHR maintenance and ongoing use once the EHR is implemented;

- ▶ Manage the vendor payment process based on successful implementation;

- ▶ Learn the importance of managing unexpected challenges and problems;

- ▶ Understand the importance of assessing how well the implementation is going (and terminating the process if necessary); and

- ▶ Prepare for the ongoing process of maintenance and enhancement, such as system upgrades, data access (by patients and health professionals), and benefits realization, after the initial implementation is completed.

▶ Converting Data from the Old System and Testing

Chapter 7, Planning and Initiating an EHR Implementation, discussed planning for the data conversion and testing the data conversion plan. The data conversion process usually begins just prior to or with the beginning of the implementation. No matter which of the several options for data conversion you select (see Chapter 7), it is very important to support the data conversion until it is completed for all legacy patient records.

The implementation team should monitor the converted records to assure that the number of total patient records in the EHR equals the number of converted legacy records to date plus the records of new patients seen since the implementation began. If these numbers do not match, there are two possible causes: Some of the old patient records have not been converted into the system and/or new EHR records have been created for patients for whom legacy records exist but have not been converted. It is far easier to identify and resolve these discrepancies early in the implementation than to discover them and have to take corrective action several weeks later.

Another testing process you can use to verify that records are in the EHR and readily available is to monitor the process of posting lab results to the EHR patient records for lab orders generated with the EHR. If this process is going smoothly with a 100 percent match, it is likely that all of the records that should have been converted are in the EHR (for example, identified by an EHR record locator as part of the order), whether electronic data interface, scanning, or key entry was the process used. But if, for example, the lab results data are not matched to patients in the EHR, there is a problem either with the record conversion setup or with matching patient lab results to EHR records.

Exhibit 8.1 shows a checklist sample for the major implementation activities.

EXHIBIT 8.1 **Implementation Plan Sample Checklist** 0010001100

IMPLEMENTATION ITEM	RESPONSIBLE PARTY	COMPLETION DATE
1. Implementation plan completion and approval		
2. Data conversion		
3. Final testing		
4. Training		
5. End-user support		
6. Checklist of milestones for vendor payments		
7. Issues log and meetings schedule with the vendor		
8. Phase-out of existing legacy applications		

Reprinted with permission, Boundary Information Group

▶ Managing the Phase-Out of the Old Applications

With an EHR implementation, some legacy electronic or paper applications may need to be phased out as they are replaced by the EHR. Examples of these include:

- ▶ The appointment scheduling system if it was in the practice management system (PMS) and is now in the EHR;

- ▶ Transcription services (might not be totally eliminated but will be significantly reduced);

- ▶ Independent electronic repositories for laboratory results, radiology reports, and so forth; and

- ▶ Paper charts and paper "shadow" charts.

Usually the phase-out of any clinical data applications provides for moving the data to the EHR through a Health Level Seven® (HL7®) or other interface so that the data resides in the EHR. Once this happens, you can take the independent data repository application offline.

A similar approach can be used for the transcription service archives if the transcription service is being eliminated and/or it is feasible to move the legacy documents to the EHR. If not, then the transcription service application will remain active, although perhaps used at a lower level, which means that the maintenance on some of the user licenses can be discontinued.

Appointment scheduling may not be a phase-out application. Virtually all group practices implementing EHRs already have an appointment scheduling system as part of their PMSs. Some EHR applications allow the continuation of the appointment scheduling system in the PMS, in which case there is no data conversion or phase-out. However, some EHRs either require or work better with the appointment scheduling and resource scheduling activities conducted within the EHR. If this is the case for your implementation, then the appointment scheduling application can be phased out after all appointments are being scheduled in the EHR and the data for the appointments that were scheduled in the PMS have been moved over (usually re-keyed) into the EHR. Again, the savings here may be the maintenance fees associated with user licenses for the appointment scheduling application. Sometimes the maintenance fees are not separable between the billing application and the appointment scheduling application.

When the EHR implementation is complete, use of paper charts should be discontinued. An EHR implementation that includes most physicians and other clinicians, but not all of them, is incomplete. "Shadow" charts, which are often used in large practices where department personnel keep departmental "partial" charts, should be discontinued with the EHR. Shadow charts are often rationalized when the real chart cannot often be found because it is in another department. With an EHR, however, all authorized users have access to the EHR records simultaneously as needed.

Another phase-out application that may occur from an EHR implementation is an independent data warehouse or repository. With the implementation of the EHR, especially if the accounts receivable and other billing information is included in a combined EHR clinical data repository (CDR), separate spreadsheets, databases, and other ad hoc analysis data sets should be reviewed to see if they can be phased out of operation. The largest benefit here is usually associated with not having to re-key the data for analysis purposes, which increases staff productivity.

To achieve some of the benefits that you defined early on in the EHR process, you need to review those applications and functions that can now be discontinued, and then phase them out to improve productivity and save the cost of maintaining applications that are no longer needed. If you have included the implementation of a PMS as part of your EHR process, the most significant phase-out challenge that you face involves the accounts receivable active and history files. The scope of options and selection of a strategy for this phase-out is beyond the scope of this book; however, you should pay significant attention to this process to preserve the accounts receivable assets of the group practice as the old accounts receivable continue to be worked for collections.

▶ Building Historical Data Prior to Going Live

In some cases, it is feasible and helpful to build historical data prior to going live. If 100 percent of the old paper charts have been scanned at the time of implementation, then all of the historical medical records data are available. The electronic data available historically are usually limited, however. For example, some physician practices have populated the EHR with transcribed dictation. One of the steps that can be taken to assist in the process in advance of implementation is to begin putting file names on the transcribed documents that include the date of the visit, the patient name, and/or a patient identifier. If this is done as the EHR selection process is under way, then six months' to a year's worth of historical dictated documents can be converted fairly easily into the EHR. (Note that this is not the same as converting the full patient chart, but it does provide for these historical records to be accessed from the day of implementation, which can be a benefit to the practice.)

Another historical data conversion process that some vendors use, if desired by the practice, is to start populating lab results data from electronic feeds (if available) into the EHR. To do this, patient records must be established for each patient (which in some cases is done by utilizing data in the PMS). This provides access to historical laboratory results through the EHR and presents the opportunity to utilize these results for trend analysis of laboratory data over a longer history than one that starts with the actual implementation.

These options, which may be supported by your vendor, have the potential to provide access to electronic historical data quicker than waiting for the complete EHR implementation. Many organizations find these electronic historical data conversion approaches to be useful, but others prefer instead to focus resources on the medical records conversion plan.

▶ Phasing in the Implementation by Facility Location or Department

To the extent that it is feasible, you should consider phasing in the EHR by facility location or by department. Medical groups with multiple locations usually phase in the EHR one location at a time, especially if individual patients tend to be seen at only one location. If individual patients are seen at multiple locations, this process becomes more difficult to manage and may not be practical. Another approach to phased-in implementation, which works well in multi-specialty practices, is to implement the EHR one department at a time. Again, though, if patients tend to be seen in multiple departments, this approach may not be feasible. Hospitals, especially inpatient hospital operations, also are not usually good candidates for a phased-in approach to EHR implementation.

There are several reasons for you to phase in the EHR. First, the phase-in provides a use test. If a small group of providers use the EHR for a few weeks, any flaws in the system, data conversion, training, and work flow should become apparent. These problems can then often be easily fixed with an impact on a minimal number of staff and patient records. Second, the implementation team that is assigned to address data conversion, technology issues, training, and operational problems can focus its attention and efforts on one department at a time or one location at a time. Also, you can set an example for others to follow. If you choose as the first one or two departments or locations those with "physician champions" and clinical staff who are enthusiastic about the EHR implementation, it is more likely that they will prove to their colleagues that they can make the EHR work and that it can be beneficial to everyone.

The time from initial operation to completion of each implementation phase is normally a few weeks to a month. However, this time frame can vary significantly, based on the organization, size, and level of readiness prior to the implementation, among other factors. If you use the same implementation team for the phase-in of each department or location, they will become more adept at performing these activities and be able to address some of the issues before the next facility or department phase-in begins.

Sometimes, however, the phased-in approach is not practical, as discussed above. If the entire enterprise, or a substantial portion of it, needs to be implemented simultaneously, two management techniques are recommended to minimize the risk of failure or significant business interruption. The first is to test every aspect of the implementation quite thoroughly, including the interoperability of the EHR between departments and locations. The second technique is to utilize a pilot or two for some of the initial production work with the EHR. Many of the significant problems that occur in the EHR implementation occur within the first week. If these can be detected and corrected without disrupting the enterprise, the smoother the rest of the implementation will proceed.

If your entire enterprise needs to be implemented essentially simultaneously, your implementation plan must include allocating the additional vendor, staff, and consultant resources to support this effort, including training, problem solving, and other functions.

▶ Training and Support

Training and support resources are crucial during the EHR implementation. Training should begin shortly before implementation. All of the clinicians and other staff who will use the EHR need to be trained on how to access and record information in the EHR, including the security controls that you have implemented. Training may be conducted in person in a classroom setting, in person on a one-on-one basis, through computer-based training, and/or with written materials for individual learning. Be sure your training program tells users what to do when they are "stuck," either because they don't know what to do next or the system is not functioning according to expectations.

It is especially important for you to provide support to the clinicians while they are seeing patients during the early implementation. You should consider developing a scenario that the clinicians can use if they are with patients and do not know what to do and need to seek help. This could be as simple as the clinicians explaining to their patients that they have just received notification via computer that there is an urgent call they need to respond to, and they will be back in a few minutes. (Be sure to emphasize the importance of clinicians either taking the portable computer with them or logging off the desktop before leaving the examining room or office.) The clinicians should know how to contact support immediately, whether it be the on-site implementation staff, the EHR support lead at his/her location, or the help desk. For each alternative, you need to be sure that adequate support is available immediately to keep the clinicians performing their job functions throughout the day. The amount of support that you need depends on many factors, including:

- ▶ Ease of use in your work flow design;
- ▶ Quality of your training program and attendance;
- ▶ Quality of the data conversion;
- ▶ Quality of the technical installation of your EHR; and
- ▶ Degree to which the clinicians have become familiar with general personal computer (PC) operation prior to the EHR implementation.

If, in planning for your training, you discover that members of your workforce are neither familiar nor comfortable with using PCs, then, prior to implementation, offer introductory training on how to use a PC with basic functionality to those who be be utilizing the EHR. In all of your job descriptions for positions that will utilize the EHR, require PC skills prior to employment or acquisition of these skills during the first week of employment, either through training offered by your organization or from an outside training provider.

The need for training and support will never disappear. Training is an ongoing process. You will always have EHR training support issues, especially with new employees and upgrades to the EHR. You will need to develop an approach to training that works for your organization and is consistent with your vendor's philosophy toward EHR upgrades. Ongoing responsibility for EHR training in most cases will be either with your overall training function (often found in large group practices) or with your EHR management team.

▶ Staffing the EHR Maintenance and Ongoing Use

Several examples of ongoing EHR-related projects are discussed in this chapter. These projects, or ones similar to them, as well as the maintenance of the EHR software and hardware upgrades and training for new personnel (and retraining existing users on any changes associated with upgrades), are likely to require a significant dedicated set of resources over an extended period of time. Therefore, do not consider the completion of the EHR selection and implementation project to be an opportunity to totally disband your EHR team. Maintain a combination of technology, work flow, and user experts as part of the team. The team can provide a core set of skills not only to plan and manage the maintenance, upgrades, and changes that occur, but also to maintain current knowledge on EHRs in general so they can provide advice to the practice's leadership on expanding EHR capabilities and new business opportunities. Be sure to budget for travel and conference fees for this team to participate in ongoing EHR vendor user conferences and industry learning experiences that will provide guidance and information to them.

▶ Managing Expected Challenges and Addressing Problems

EHR selection and implementation is complex. The initial implementation of the EHR into production is perhaps the most sensitive and one of the most critical components of the overall project because the clinicians and patients are directly involved. Therefore, you want to have invested significant resources in preparing, testing, and training to minimize the disruptions that occur. However, because the EHR implementation involves people, cultural change, technology, and often data flows involving other vendor products, you should expect that there will be deviations from the implementation plan. These deviations may be caused by technology, human beings, unaccounted-for scenarios, and data errors, among other factors.

Some of the problem issues that have existed for a long time in your practice operation may become visible to the clinicians for the first time because they now have direct electronic access to the records. For instance, many practices spend considerable resources each day making sure that all the information that is supposed to be in the paper chart is there before the physician sees the patient the next day. With an EHR, much of that extra work activity is eliminated – or can be, if the right work flow structure has been put in place. For instance, if certain referral documentation is needed before new patients can be seen, and the pattern when documentation is missing has been for staff to call the referring physician or hospital the day before to request it be faxed for inclusion into the new patient chart, then that process will not disappear just because you have implemented an EHR.

What can be changed, though, is the work flow so an automated checklist and alerts are provided to the appropriate staff person regarding specific documents that are missing and need to be acquired and added to the EHR prior to the scheduled appointment. These document requests can then be processed days earlier, if desired.

Most of the problems that can occur are unpredictable, but with so many possibilities, you can expect some events to happen that are not expected. Therefore, you should have a plan to manage the unexpected when it occurs. The plan can include a first response by the onsite implementation team, or you may choose to create a "war room" if you have implemented an entire enterprise at one time. With this latter strategy, you need to inform everyone involved about what to do and how to contact the war room when problems occur. It is also important that, as problems are resolved, the resolution be communicated to all the affected parties, as well as those who might become affected. In this way, they will know the issue has been addressed or that you are working on a resolution, and there is a "workaround" that they should use in the meantime.

Most of the time, the significant challenges occur during the first few days or weeks of implementation, especially if you have prepared well with the steps described in Chapter 7, Planning and Initiating an EHR Implementation. If your vendor team is not on site during the implementation, you need to arrange a process for them to escalate your problems for resolution quickly during this crucial period.

▶ Contingency Planning

Having a contingency plan for every information system is a good business practice. It is also a requirement for Health Insurance Portability and Accountability Act (HIPAA) Security Rule compliance (after April 21, 2005) for all providers who are HIPAA-covered entities.[1] One option for a contingency plan during the implementation is to maintain the paper charts, transcriptions, and other records after they are converted for a period of several months or longer in an easily accessible place.

A second option for the contingency plan for EHR implementation failure may be to utilize the capability (if it exists) within the EHR to create an equivalent paper medical record that can be used when patients request paper copies of their medical records or that copies be sent to another provider. Rather than routinely printing out all of these records after each new record entry, investigate whether it is possible to electronically save the print image of each patient's record in this format on a separate server, where it can be printed or electronically accessed on an as-needed basis through a commonly used software program, such as Microsoft Word® or a browser.

Another component of the contingency plan is to have an alternative methodology for processing patients if the EHR system fails either during implementation or subsequently. This plan could include temporarily using a paper-based process to record new patient data, while accessing existing patient data through the second option above (paper record). This component is consistent with the HIPAA Security Rule contingency plan requirement.[2]

▶ Clinical Database Use to Improve Quality of Care and Business Operations

If your EHR includes a CDR that is automatically populated with orders, results, and your clinical document information, you can analyze the data in new ways. For instance, if there is a drug recall, you can search the database quickly to identify and contact the patients who have been prescribed the specific drug involved (see the 50-physician practice example in Chapter 7). You can program alerts to remind the clinicians during their next encounters with certain patients of activities that are not being followed (e.g., not refilling prescriptions for chronic conditions, which may mean that the patient is not compliant with taking the prescribed medication). You can search the database for patients who are beyond the recommended time for their next mammogram or prostate-specific antigen (PSA) test, and then process them through your scheduling staff.

The clinical data repository can also be used to review and educate physicians on their performance. For instance, the database can compare drug prescribing patterns among physicians for patients with the same illness or condition, together with patient outcomes, to learn which prescribing patterns work best. The outcome measurements may include weight loss, blood pressure readings, or laboratory results, all of which are quantifiable and measurable. These are but a few examples of new data analysis capabilities that are relatively inexpensive as a secondary benefit of the EHR.

▶ Patient Access to Clinical Data

Providing patient access to clinical data may be one of your primary objectives in implementing the EHR, or it may be considered as a secondary or lesser implementation, if at all. Increasingly, physician practices are providing access to patients over the Internet for a variety of functions, including appointment requests and access to clinical and patient education information. With appropriate security controls, many EHR vendor products include the capability (either with the EHR license or as an additional licensed product) to present patients with electronic access to their own data. Some practices are limiting data access to lab results, whereas others are providing a variety of clinical information to patients. As you consider providing patient access to clinical information, you need to take into account the HIPAA Privacy and Security requirements.

Just as you spent significant time customizing the work flow and data presentation templates for your clinicians (see Chapter 7), you should consider how patients approach the access and use of their own data by helping them design a personal health record (PHR). Many practices are doing this by providing access to a portion of (or summary from) the EHR. Such an electronic patient health record (EPHR) can be an important benefit for patients and the practice itself.

The EPHR implementation may include a patient registration process. In providing this, you should offer e-mail and/or telephone support for patients who are having difficulty registering or accessing their own data. You may also choose to provide the same patient access at kiosks in your practice settings. Another benefit to consider providing to patients is educational material related to their specific conditions and concerns, either through electronic library products that supply patient education information or your own material.

Exhibit 8.2 presents a list of potential online functions for EPHRs that you may consider for your practice. Three of the major potential benefits for implementing some or all of these functions include:

> ▶ EPHRs can increase staff productivity and data accuracy by having the patient complete an electronic registration with edits, which modifies the patient record with changes in demographic information and insurance. This reduces staff time to key the data and staff time at the check-in desk when registering new patients.

▶ Health assessments can also be captured as part of an EPHR – often providing more complete information than what is usually captured during a relatively short visit.

▶ EPHRs may increase patient compliance with medications and/or monitoring illnesses by providing patients access to their own information (e.g., lab results), as well as patient education materials on a 24/7 basis. Medication reconciliation may be enhanced by having each patient record medications (including OTC and herbal supplements) in his/her EHR that can be reviewed and validated during subsequent visits.

▶ EPHRs reduce the number of telephone calls for scheduling appointments and prescription refills. The work can be processed without calling the patient back by using a more efficient process and responding electronically.

Although security and privacy concerns are associated with allowing patient access to this information, there are several options where this communication can be deployed consistent with the requirements of the HIPAA Privacy and Security Rules. Several case studies of physician practices and hospitals deploying one or more of these functions to patients are described in *Connecting for Health: A Public-Private Collaborative.*[3]

EXHIBIT 8.2   Potential Online Functions for EPHRs   000100011001

FUNCTION	CHECK (✔) IF INCLUDED IN YOUR APPLICATION
1. Initial registration	
2. Changes in registration	
3. Appointment request	
4. Prescription refill request	
5. Patient education information request	
6. Lab results	
7. Selected EHR sections/views	
8. Full patient access to his/her EHR information	

Reprinted with permission, Boundary Information Group

One other area to be addressed in setting up an EPHR is liability. Any website or USB storage device used for EHR should clearly and carefully establish parameters for use. For example, an EPHR is not a substitute for a personal appointment or visit, especially in the case of an emergency, when patients should be directed to call 9-1-1 or the practice's emergency phone number. If an interactive Web site is offered, patients should clearly understand that a response will take a certain amount of time (e.g., 24, 48, or 72 hours). Finally, if the EPHR permits the patient to compile information from other providers or notes written by the patient, the practice should explain its policy on if and when such information may be reviewed. It may be wise to have legal counsel review such advice.

▶ Exchanging Your Data with Other Physician Practices and Providers

The health care industry in the United States is moving toward a process by which health information can easily be exchanged electronically among providers. But it is not there yet. There are two major barriers to achieving this exchange. One is the lack of clinical data element standards with standard nomenclature and definitions for the patient record. The U.S. Department of Health and Human Services (HHS) is currently working on developing a core set of mandatory electronic medical record (EMR) data elements that will have standard definitions and nomenclature so that data can be exchanged among providers.

The second major barrier is that we do not yet have a standard patient identifier. Such a standard identifier was specified in the administrative simplification provisions of HIPAA in 1996. However, the U.S. Congress has decided since 1996 to not allow any funding for the development of the standard patient identifier until good privacy protection is in place. The implementation of the HIPAA Privacy Rule in 2003 may now provide sufficient privacy protections in place to consider a unique patient identifier.

Whereas some health care industry organizations are supportive of this approach, others are against it due to privacy concerns. Without a unique patient identifier, the issue of identifying who the data belong to when they arrive at a provider's "electronic doorstep" becomes difficult and complex, unless the data are being sent in response to an inquiry from a requesting provider and include an identifying number that can be used in the response. For instance, if the physician orders an X-ray from the hospital and the hospital sends back the results of the X-ray, the order and response could both have an identifying number that would be recognizable to the physician's practice and could be used to properly place the results in the appropriate patient record in the EHR. In contrast, if the patient goes to the emergency room (ER) in the hospital and an X-ray is taken, and the patient while in the ER requests that a copy of the radiology report be sent to his/her primary care physician, the hospital would not know the internal identifying number for that patient in the physician practice. Having a unique and universal patient identifier would solve that problem.

Demonstration projects in several areas around the nation will provide the basis for the industry to move in a direction where either a unique patient identifier is used, or another alternative reasonable approach is developed. Two demonstration projects that have moved forward very aggressively are located in Indianapolis, Ind. and Santa Barbara, Calif. From such demonstrations, the health care industry will learn how to best approach a changeover during a transition period that may last several years.

▶ Benefits Realization

At the start of the EHR selection and planning process, you developed a list of benefits and a return on investment (ROI) model for your practice. Once the implementation has been completed, it is important to measure your organization's performance against the benefits that were projected. You may find that some of the expenditures that were targeted for reduction with the EHR are still occurring, as duplicate work and record-keeping efforts, because the staff are reluctant to let go of the legacy work flow instead of relying on the EHR. It may also be the case that the work flow needs to be changed to achieve the benefits or that some of the alerts or decision support capabilities were not turned on (or were turned off) to initially simplify the learning process. It is possible that some of the projected benefits cannot be realized without changing the technology and culture of the organization.

A benefits review is important on an ongoing basis. In fact, it is appropriate to add new benefit goals when considering expanding the capabilities of the EHR to e-prescribing, EPHR, and other projects. For instance, both e-prescribing and EPHR could reduce the number of telephone calls to the practice.

Importantly, by measuring your achieved benefits against your projections and revising the benefits realization model as further investments are made in the EHR, you can assure your group practice that it will realize the benefits of the EHR.

▶ Planning for EHR Upgrades

During your EHR selection process, your vendor documented its history of upgrades, including frequency. Because most EHR vendors continue to add to their product capabilities and scope, you can expect that there will be upgrades available for your EHR on at least an annual basis for the next several years. Although it is best to minimize upgrade activity just before and during implementation, once the implementation is completed you should plan on reviewing software upgrades available from your vendor and begin a process of implementing upgrade capabilities on an ongoing basis. The frequency of upgrades and their scope will have an impact on your staffing requirements. In some cases, upgrades may require additional staff training, or offer functions that you may not need.

Upgrades can also involve hardware. You may need to add data storage capacity after a period of time when you have built up a significant inventory of EHRs. There may be new hardware devices for users and for the EHR infrastructure that your organization will find attractive because either they work better for the end user or they are more reliable. Your network infrastructure should be monitored for performance (e.g., reliability, response time) and, if necessary, upgraded to meet your performance standards.

▶ Planning for Use of National Clinical Data Standards

As of the end of 2004, no clinical data standards are either mandated by the federal government or accepted uniformly throughout the industry. The industry can expect, though, that there will be some form of government and/or industry recognition and adoption of national clinical data standards in the future. Among the federal government activities that you should monitor for these national clinical data standards are the following (see also Chapter 9, The EHR Regulatory and Standards Environment):

> ▶ National Committee on Vital and Health Statistics (NCVHS). Refer to the Feb. 27, 2002, letter to the secretary of HHS regarding recommendations for the first set of patient medical record information (PMRI) standards.[4]

▶ The Centers for Medicare and Medicaid Services (CMS). CMS is expected to issue the electronic claims attachment HIPAA standard transaction as a Notice of Proposed Rule Making (NPRM) in 2005. The clinical data standards for the transaction are defined by HL7.[5]

▶ The Consolidated Health Initiative (CHI), which is part of the Federal e-gov initiative. Several data and messaging standards have been adopted for use by federal government agencies including the Systematized Nomenclature of Medicine (SNOMED®) and HL7 messaging standards.[6]

▶ E-prescribing transactions specification. This specification is expected from CMS, and HHS is likely to endorse the SCRIPT transaction standard from NCPDP for Medicare Part D prescriptions sent from providers to retail and community pharmacies.[7]

In the future, either through federal requirements or industry adoption by consensus, standardization of some of the clinical data used in EHRs is likely. By utilizing the data standards in the transactions (e.g., electronic claims attachment and e-prescribing), providers will minimize the need for "translators" to convert internal EHR data to be used in transactions to other providers and health plans and be well positioned to communicate clinical data electronically to other providers and health plans.

▶ Vendor Payments Tied to Implementation Milestones

If your vendor payment schedule is tied to implementation milestones, you need to evaluate your implementation progress to the milestone payment criteria. There may have been previous milestones for payments based on delivery, loading of software for testing, and so forth. If one or more milestones are associated with implementation, these need to be reviewed and monitored during the implementation project.

If you use a payment milestone of first productive use or within 30 days of first productive use, you will be required to make the appropriate payment to the vendor per your contract based on when the first clinician productively uses the EHR to treat a patient, refills a prescription, or some other use criterion. Usually, the way these contractual terms are written, it doesn't matter whether one user or a hundred users are productively utilizing the system to trigger the first productive use payment. If continuous use for 30 days is included in the payment criteria, then it is extremely important that if things are not going well due to responsibilities of the vendor, and the difficulties are not being addressed promptly, to come to terms with the vendor in writing before the 30 days are up. You may agree either to shut down the use of the EHR or to defer the milestone payment until the problems are corrected to your satisfaction.

You also may have a payment milestone associated with full implementation and use of all functions. You and the vendor should agree to a written checklist to document this milestone. This list is your last financial leverage point with the vendor if you have not been able to fully implement everything that was contracted.

Likewise, if you have utilized incentive payments for the EHR contract, these criteria must also be monitored during the implementation. Incentive payments are often based not only on time, but on performance, so it is extremely important to document events as they occur – for example, if the vendor or your organization has not provided product or resources when scheduled or has failed to address an identified problem within a reasonable time frame. This documentation should be reviewed on an ongoing basis from the time of contract signing until full implementation is completed. That way, the vendor and your management will be aware of any identified problems and how they are being addressed as well as those that are not being addressed in a timely fashion.

The reason for including incentive clauses in EHR contracts is primarily not to create penalties and profits, but rather to create a mutual aligned structure for the vendor and provider to work collaboratively toward successfully implementing a complex project. This can work well only if both parties agree to document and resolve issues as they arise to the best of their abilities and to help each other work toward the collaborative goal. Sometimes these issues can be resolved only by elevating the issue to a higher authority within the vendor or provider organization to allocate the resources or make the decisions to support the contract and implementation plan. If you are unfamiliar with operating in this type of relationship with a vendor, use outside consultant resources to provide the management, documentation, and resolution skills needed to work out problems and keep the project moving forward.

Finally, when the implementation has successfully been completed, recognize this as a special event because it will have taken the work efforts of most of your workforce and a significant number of resources from the vendor. A celebration is appropriate in a style and at a level that is consistent with your organization's philosophy and culture. The vendor team should be included in this celebration because the two organizations will have worked so closely together over a long period to achieve this success.

▶ Knowing When to Pull the Plug on a Project Gone Bad

Occasionally, information systems and work flow changes as complex as the EHR do not go as planned, and the problems are not easily resolved. When this happens there are usually one or more sources of problems that cannot be easily corrected, such as:

- ▶ The data conversion is not working;

- ▶ Staff are either not trained well enough or not motivated to use the EHR correctly;

- ▶ The technology fails, including working too slowly to support productive use;

- ▶ The data, once entered, are not being managed properly by the EHR application;

- ▶ Critical interfaces fail; or

- ▶ The vendor no longer supports or refuses to support the product.

When one or more significant issues occur that cannot be readily fixed or accommodated, no matter what the root cause, the leadership responsible for the EHR must make a decision or recommendation to executive management to limit the scope of the implementation until the problems are resolved or, in an extreme case, to abandon the project. This is not an easy decision, considering all of the resources and planning that have occurred throughout the organization. However, in rare circumstances, it is the appropriate action to take. Although no guidelines exist for when such action is appropriate, the EHR leadership must understand that failure can happen, and if it does, these leaders are the ones responsible for making the decision to limit or stop the project.

Many of the planning issues described in Chapter 7 will minimize the chances of failure. The recommendation at the end of that chapter to not move forward with the implementation until all of your planned testing has been conducted successfully is a further step to assure that there is at most a minimum chance that you will be faced with this decision.

▶ Conclusion

The purpose of all of the planning steps described in Chapter 7 was to pre-pare for a successful implementation with minimum problems. This chap-ter has discussed the need to be able to adapt the recommendations for the implementation and your collective resources to best meet the needs of your organization as the implementation occurs. It is crucial to continu-ously monitor the implementation to make sure it is going smoothly and to address issues as they occur. Once the EHR is fully implemented, those applications no longer needed should be discontinued, which can be accomplished by appropriate data transfers. Vendor payments associated with implementation milestones should be made consistent with the terms of your contract.

The EHR "project" isn't over when the implementation is complete, however. Resources are needed on an ongoing basis to support upgrades to the software and hardware utilized in the EHR as well as to expand the functionality of the EHR. Consider maintaining a core EHR team representing the key stake-holders in your organization who will maintain management responsibility for enhancements and updates as well as be responsible for monitoring EHR activities nationally and in medical groups similar to your own practice.

NOTES

1. *Federal Register,* February 20, 2003, pp 8377-8378.
2. *Ibid.* Paper forms may be used to schedule appointments, register patients, document clinical findings, place orders, and conduct other business until the system is restored. This may be your control for emergency mode operation.
3. Markle Foundation, *Connecting for Health: A Public-Private Collaborative*, The Personal Health Working Group Final Report, July 1, 2003 (www.connectingforhealth.org/resources/generalresources.html).
4. See the National Committee on Vital Health and Statistics Web site (www.ncvhs.dhhs.gov).
5. See the Centers for Medicare and Medicaid Web site (www.cms.hhs.gov); see also the Health Level Seven" Web site (www.hl7.org/) for information on HL7.
6. Monitor the adoption of CHI standards for federal government agencies at the official Web site of President's E-Government Initiative (www.whitehouse.gov/omb/egov/gtob/health_informatics.htm).
7. See the National Council for Prescription Drug Program Web site (www.ncpdp.org). For the list of recommended e-prescribing standards as recommended by the NCVHS, go to the National Committee on Vital Health and Statistics Web site (www.ncvhs.hhs.gov).

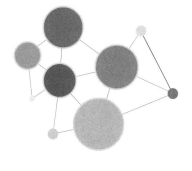

► N I N E

The EHR Regulatory and Standards Environment

"Our 21st century health care system
uses a 19th century paperwork system"

– President George W. Bush, April 27, 2004

Once you have implemented an EHR in your practice, your work is far from being done. Legislation and initiatives regarding standards are evolving in regard to this relatively new environment. Federal regulatory and non-regulatory initiatives as well as several pending industry standards will influence the use of medical data and messaging and the functional characteristics of EHRs in the coming years. By monitoring the relevant organizations and agencies, you can keep abreast of the latest developments. Use the information in this chapter to assure that your practice is informed of available EHR resources. Other sources of EHR information include EHR vendors and associations such as the Medical Group Management Association (MGMA) and the physician specialty societies.

THIS CHAPTER IDENTIFIES the types of organizations you should monitor regarding the EHR regulatory and standards environment. Specifically, this chapter helps you:

► Monitor the relevant sources of information to keep abreast of changes; and

▶ Identify some of the more important types of information available from an EHR perspective (highlighted in the EHR tracking issues listed for each source).

Health care leaders in both government and private industry are calling for the adoption of critical standards and the development of heath information exchanges, primarily through local initiatives termed Regional Health Information Organizations (RHIOs). These RHIOs will form a comprehensive knowledge-based network of interoperable systems (including EHRs in hospitals and practices) that will be capable of providing critical health information for sound clinical decisions whenever and wherever needed. This vision of a transformed health care system includes communication networks, message and content standards, computer applications, and confidentiality protections, as well as widespread utilization of EHR in ambulatory settings. In addition, several health insurance companies are currently offering incentives to physicians to implement and use EHRs.

Track the federal government entities, standards development organizations, and associations described in this chapter for developments that impact EHRs. These sources are continually developing new information on EHRs; their Web sites will keep you current on EHR information.

▶ Federal Government Programs

The federal government has been looking increasingly to technology for solutions to the many problems associated with the inefficiencies of the health care system. At both the congressional and administrative levels, lawmakers are seeking potential avenues to facilitate the adoption of EHR. Several members of the 108th Congress introduced legislation seeking financial incentives for providers to move forward with health technology. Although none of these bills became law, it is clear that the movement to support EHR is gaining considerable strength on Capitol Hill. On the administrative side, the U.S. Department of Health and Human Services (HHS) is actively promoting health technology by developing demonstration programs, allocating some grant monies to providers to migrate to EHR, and actively supporting industry efforts to develop standards and educate the provider community to the benefits of these systems.

Office of the National Health Information Technology Coordinator
www.hhs.gov/healthit

One of the catalysts for the move to health information technology (HIT) will certainly be the HHS Office of the National Health Information Technology Coordinator (ONCHIT). On April 27, 2004, President George W. Bush announced an executive order establishing ONCHIT as a new sub-cabinet-level agency and called for most Americans to have a computerized health record within 10 years. The president also identified key health care leaders to attend a national summit to discuss how best to move forward with HIT.

> ### EHR Tracking Issues for ONCHIT
>
> ► Incentives for EHR adoption
>
> ► Regional collaborations to interconnect clinicians
>
> ► Personal health records
>
> ► Public health record reporting and research

At this summit, HHS Secretary Tommy Thompson introduced David J. Brailer as the first HIT coordinator. Shortly after his appointment, Brailer issued a report aligning a strategic framework for a new vision of health care made possible through the use of IT – strategic actions embraced by the public and private health sectors that need to be taken over many years. The four major goals are:

- ► *Goal 1:* Inform clinical practice, which includes creating incentives for EHR adoption and reducing risk of EHR investment while promoting EHR diffusion in rural and underserved areas.

- ► *Goal 2:* Interconnect clinicians, which includes fostering regional collaborations, developing a national health information network, and coordinating the federal health information systems.

- ► *Goal 3:* Personalize care, including encouraging the use of personal health records (PHRs), enhancing informed consumer choice, and promoting use of telehealth systems.

- ► *Goal 4:* Improve population health, including the strategies of unifying public health surveillance architectures, streamlining quality and health status monitoring, and accelerating research and dissemination of evidence.

Monitor activities of this office for the role of EHRs in achieving these goals. As stated on the ONCHIT Web site, at the time of ONCHIT's establishment, an important aspect of the initiative to promote EHRs was "the development of a nationwide interoperable health information technology infrastructure that can facilitate improvements in safety, quality, efficiency, and care coordination

---

0010100101101001010010100100

EHR Tracking Issues for AHRQ

- ▶ National Guideline Clearinghouse™ (www.guideline.gov)

- ▶ National Quality Measures Clearinghouse™

- ▶ National Health Information Technology Resource Center

- ▶ Quality assessment reports (medical errors and patient safety reports, national health care quality and disparities reports, and evidence-based practice center reports)

- ▶ Outcomes and effectiveness research findings for clinicians

- ▶ Funding opportunities for adoption of health information technology

- ▶ EHR case studies and lessons learned from research projects

---

Agency for Healthcare Research and Quality
www.ahrq.gov

The Agency for Healthcare Research and Quality (AHRQ) is an organization that funds health services research and demonstration programs. Its focus is clinical, including evidence-based practice, outcomes and effectiveness of care, technology assessment, preventive services, and clinical practice guidelines. Monitor this organization for research and demonstration funding activities as well as the knowledge base that it has developed and published (e.g., the National Guideline Clearinghouse™, which provides online information on clinical practice guidelines, and the National Quality Measures Clearinghouse™, an online database of health care quality measures). Its funding has included and is likely to continue to include many initiatives associated with EHRs and the exchange of clinical data among provider organizations. On October 13, 2004, for example, AHRQ announced $139 million in grants and contracts to promote the use of HIT.

National Health Information Infrastructure
www.aspe.hhs.gov/sp.nhii

The National Health Information Infrastructure (NHII) was formed to focus on the federal government initiatives associated with developing a comprehensive knowledge-base network that would support the exchange of information among health care providers, public health workers, and others with interoperable systems and technology standards. Many of the topics addressed by the NHII at its conferences and other activities concern the direct or indirect use of EHRs with a particular focus on how information is transmitted and shared from the provider entities to others, including those for public health purposes.

> 0010100101101001010010100100

> ### EHR Tracking Issues for NHII
>
> ► Patient safety
>
> ► Quality of care
>
> ► Cost efficiency

The focus of this program is to improve the effectiveness, efficiency, and overall quality of health and health care in the United States. Specifically, for your purposes, among other goals, the NHII seeks to improve patient safety, such as through alerts for medication errors or drug allergies; to improve health care quality, such as having complete medical records available and integrating health information from multiple sources and providers; and to better understand health care costs.

National Committee on Vital and Health Statistics
www.ncvhs.hhs.gov

The National Committee on Vital Health Statistics (NCVHS) is the HHS Statutory Public Advisory Body to the secretary of HHS on health data, statistics, and national health information policy. The committee and its subcommittees meet periodically and publish their reports and recommendations online. Check especially the Subcommittee on Standards and Security, which is charged with monitoring and making recommendations to the full committee on health data standards and security. Significant initiatives of this subcommittee involve the development of

> 0010100101101001010010100100

> ### EHR Tracking Issues for NCVHS
>
> ► e-prescribing standards
>
> ► Measuring health care quality
>
> ► Uniform standards for electronic exchange of PMRI (data comparability and interoperability)
>
> ► Privacy and security
>
> ► National health information infrastructure

recommendations for uniform data standards for patient medical record information (PMRI) and the electronic exchange of such information, including EHRs as well as recommendations regarding e-prescribing standards.

National Library of Medicine
www.nlm.nih.gov

The U.S. National Library of Medicine (NLM), the world's largest medical library, is part of the National Institutes of Health (NIH). The NLM collects materials and provides information and research services in all areas of biomedicine and health care. Use this source to keep current with new technology and information networking.

As part of compiling bibliographic material, the NLM has created the Unified Medical Language System® (UMLS®), which is a comprehensive mapping structure among medical vocabularies. For example, the NLM has mapped the Systematized Nomenclature of Medicine (SNOMED®) to the International Classification of Diseases (ICD) and the Current Procedural Terminology® (CPT®), so that in the future it may be possible to have an EHR automatically create codes needed for reimbursement (in ICD and CPT) from data entered into the EHR and encoded by the computer in SNOMED.

001010010110100101001010100100

EHR Tracking Issues for NLM

▶ SNOMED CT

▶ Mapping between SNOMED CT and other codes

▶ UMLS encompassing maps among numerous terminologies and code sets

The NLM, on behalf of HHS, has entered into an agreement with the College of American Pathologists (CAP) for a perpetual license for the core SNOMED Clinical Terms (SNOMED CT®) and its ongoing updates. The terms of this license make SNOMED CT available to U.S. users at no cost through the UMLS Metathesaurus®. SNOWMED CT is a comprehensive clinical terminology (available in Spanish and English) formed by the convergence of SNOMED RT® (Reference Terminology) and the United Kingdom National Health Service Clinical Terms Version 3. NLM is in the process of converting crosswalks between SNOMED CT and other coding structures. For more information on SNOMED CT, go to www.snomed.org; see also Chapter 2, EHR Technology, and Chapter 3, Determining Your Group's Objectives, in this book.)

For e-prescribing, the NLM, in conjunction with the FDA, is mapping the clinical drug terminology, RxNorm, that physicians would use to select drugs to the National Drug Code (NDC) used by retail pharmacies for packaged drugs.

Centers for Medicare & Medicaid Services
www.cms.hhs.gov

On July 21, 2004, the Centers for Medicare & Medicaid Services (CMS), under HHS, announced initiatives to promote the adoption of reliable, confidential EHRs, particularly in physicians' offices. CMS administrator Mark B. McClellan stated, "We are committed to using health information technology to improve health and health care not only for Medicare's 41 million beneficiaries, but for all Americans." CMS plans to conduct demonstration programs involving financial incentives for EHR adoption. Additionally, demonstration programs will determine how EHR adoption affects the quality and cost of health care.

> **EHR Tracking Issues for CMS**
> ► e-prescribing
> ► EHR with regard to Medicare

One of the many initiatives promoted by CMS is nationwide e-prescribing. CMS is reviewing existing e-prescription programs to determine what features can be adopted for the new Medicare drug benefit of the Medicare Prescription Drug, Improvement and Modernization Act (MMA) of 2003, and what incentives can make e-prescribing more attractive to physicians, whose participation in this initiative is optional.

Consolidated Health Informatics
www.whitehouse.gov/omb/egov/gtob/health_informatics.htm
or www.whitehouse.gov/omb/egov

Consolidated Health Informatics (CHI) is administered in the Office of HIPAA Standards, CMS. It involves all federal agencies that purchase and use information systems, including CMS, the Department of Veterans Affairs, and the Department of Defense. The purpose of CHI is to identify and adopt existing health information interoperability standards that can be used by all agencies in the federal

> **EHR Tracking Issues for CHI**
> ► Clinical data messaging standards
> ► Vocabulary standards
> ► SNOMED CT
> ► LOINC

government to form a common enterprise-wide business and technology infrastructure.

This initiative is part of the federal government's e-gov strategy to provide technology-based services and information on the Internet. More than twenty standards have been adopted as of October 2004, and they apply to all federal government agencies. For example, CHI not only standardizes health care data, messaging, and transactions within the federal government, it also influences the private sector by requiring vendors that supply software applications to federal government agencies to support these standards, with the anticipation that they will therefore also be supplied to the private sector. For example, the standards adopted by CHI include SNOMED CT and standardized electronic exchange of laboratory test orders, drug labels, and other clinical orders with the Logical Observation Identifier Name Codes® (LOINC®). Adopted standards were announced on March 21, 2003, and May 6, 2004.

► Standards Organizations

ASTM International
www.astm.org

ASTM International is a worldwide voluntary standards organization. It is a trusted source for technical standards for materials, products, systems, and services. The acronym is an artifact of its original name, the American Society for Testing Materials.

> **EHR Tracking Issues for ASTM**
>
> ► Clinical data definitions
>
> ► EHR content and structure
>
> ► Continuity of Care Record
>
> ► Technical specification for access controls and authentication measures

One of the ASTM standards development activities is the ASTM Committee E31 on Health Care Informatics. Check on the following ASTM subcommittees that work on EHR standards (go to www.astm.org and search for Committee E31, and then select Subcommittees and Standards):

- ► E31.01 Controlled Health Vocabularies for Healthcare Informatics
- ► E31.19 Electronic Health Record Content and Structure
- ► E31.20 Security and Privacy

- ► E31.22 Health Information Transcription and Documentation

- ► E31.23 Modeling for Health Informatics

- ► E31.28 Electronic Health Records

- ► E31.90 Executive

The E31.28 Electronic Health Records Subcommittee document WK4363, Standard Specification for the Continuity of Care Record (CCR), is a core dataset of the most relevant and timely facts about a patient's health care.

Accredited Standards Committee X12
www.X12.org or www.wpc-edi.com

In 1979, the American National Standards Institute (ANSI) chartered the Accredited Standards Committee (ASC) X12 to develop electronic data interchange (EDI) standards to support business transactions for the health care industry. The specific health care industry transactions in which you would be interested are addressed through the X12N (insurance) subcommittee, hence the reference to X12N for health care EDI transaction standards. For further information about ASC X12N, go to www.x12.org, pull down the menu under Committees/Groups, and select Subcommittee X12N. The HIPAA ASC X12N transactions implementation guides are available at www.wpc-edi.com.

> 0010100101101001010010100100
>
> **EHR Tracking Issues for ASC X12**
>
> ► Demographic data definitions
>
> ► Health care administrative data definitions
>
> ► Electronic claims attachments plans

Historically, X12N has been concerned primarily with administrative transactions. Some of the ASC X12N administrative transactions, such as eligibility inquiry and response, may be used directly from the EHR if, for example, the provider is trying to verify eligibility for a benefit through the EHR while seeing the patient. X12N serves as a liaison with Health Level 7® (HL7®; see below) to coordinate activities that relate to health insurance standards.

The ASC X12N transaction standards include demographic and other administrative definition standards that must be used in the transactions. These data definitions can be used in EHRs and other internal medical group information systems, in which case there will be a reduced need for translation of data prior to transmission to other providers and health plans. The electronic claims attachment standard developed by HL7 (discussed next) is to be transmitted between providers and health plans electronically in an ASC X12N envelope. The standard has been developed and will be included in the HIPAA required transaction standards in the future. The data used to populate the electronic claims attachment will in many cases come from the medical group's EHR.

Health Level Seven
www.hl7.org

001010010110100101001010010010

EHR Tracking Issues for HL7

▶ EHR functional descriptors model

▶ Clinical data element definitions

▶ Clinical transaction standards (e.g., HIPAA claims attachments)

▶ Clinical data messaging standards

Health Level Seven (HL7) is a Standards Developing Organization (SDO) functioning in the health care industry. This ANSI-accredited non-profit organization focuses on interface standards within health care organizations. HL7 uses a process within its structure to promote the fastest feasible development of standards that are both responsive and responsible. The group continues to dedicate its efforts to ensuring concurrence with other U.S. and international standards development activities throughout the world.

A substantial part of HL7's activities concern the transmission of clinical and administrative data. The HL7 mission statement states that it exists "to provide standards for the exchange, management and integration of data that support clinical patient care and the management, delivery and evaluation of healthcare services."

HL7 and ASC X12 have been working together to standardize the content of various health care claims attachments, in response to HIPAA administrative simplification regulations. For the six recommended claims attachment standards that are in the process of being introduced, go to www.hl7.org and choose HIPAA from the menu, or go to the Washington Publishing Company Web site www.wpc-edi.com and select HIPAA.

HL7 has also developed an EHR functional model and standard. For information about the HL7 EHR functional model and standard, go to "About HL7" on www.hl7.org, and choose Electronic Health Record from the menu.

National Council for Prescription Drug Programs
www.ncpdp.org

The National Council for Prescription Drug Programs, Inc. (NCPDP) is a not-for-profit ANSI-accredited SDO representing virtually every sector of the pharmacy services industry. NCPDP transaction standards are designed for real-time processing. Claims, eligibility and remittance advice are examples of electronic NCPDP transactions standards used

> 0010100101101001010010100100
>
> ### EHR Tracking Issues for NCPDP
>
> ▶ Demographic and clinical data definitions for the pharmacy services sector
>
> ▶ SCRIPT standard

by the pharmacy services industry. Refer to the NCPDP Web site for information on standards for data transfer from and to the health care industry's pharmacy services sector.

The NCPDP SCRIPT standard has been developed for electronic data interchange of prescription transactions (e.g., new prescriptions, refills, change requests) to communicate between e-prescribing devices and retail pharmacies. It is expected to be the e-prescribing standard required by Medicare under the MMA. See Chapter 3, Determining Your Group's Objectives, and Chapter 8, Implementation and Ongoing Operations – Going Live with Your EHR, in this book for more information on the SCRIPT standard.

▶ Other Health-Related Organizations

American Health Information Management Association
www.ahima.org

The American Health Information Management Association (AHIMA) is a member organization whose purpose not only encompasses health information management but also coding and electronic health records, offering credentialing in these disciplines as well as academic program accreditation. The association sponsors the e-HIM™ (electronic health information) initiative that promotes the migration from paper records to EHR, the building

```
0010100101101001010010100100
```

EHR Tracking Issues for AHIMA

▶ Collaborative activities

▶ Best practices

▶ Body of knowledge

▶ EHR education

▶ Personal health records

of an electronic health information infrastructure, and innovation in institutional and personal medical records management to produce measurable costs and improved quality results.

The AHIMA Web site outlines a body of knowledge that focuses on EHR best practices that include core data sets for medical practice EHRs, e-mail procedures, electronic signatures, master person index maintenance, hybrid records management, and legal issues, including HIPAA guidance and medical records retention requirements.

An advocate of patient safety and personal health records, AHIMA has developed a Web site, www.myPHR.com, to educate the public about personal health records and related issues, including how to gain access to them and ensure confidentiality of personal health information.

eHealth Initiative
www.ehealthinitiative.org

```
0010100101101001010010100100
```

EHR Tracking Issues for eHealth Initiative

▶ Resource Center

▶ Grant application resources

▶ White papers and workgroups, including EHR for small and medium-sized practices and e-prescribing

▶ Funded communities for health information exchanges

eHealth Initiative and the Foundation for eHealth Initiative are nonprofit organizations whose missions are to drive improvement in the quality, safety, and efficiency of health care through information and information technology (IT).

Reports that you might find useful include Accelerating the Adoption of Computerized Prescribing in the Ambulatory Environment, which is available on the eHealth Initiative Web site under Electronic Prescribing; and Connecting for Health ... a Public-Private Collaborative Preliminary Roadmap for Achieving Electronic Connectivity in Health Care, from eHealth Initiative's Connecting Communities for Better Health Resource

Center. The Resource Center includes information on community awards totaling more than $2 million to improve connectivity, reduce medical errors, and create more efficient health care for patients. On July 1, 2004, eHealth Initiatives funded nine communities to evaluate approaches to the use of HIT, including EHRs.

eHealth Initiative has also announced the creation of Working Group for Health Information Technology in Small Practices, which will develop resources for using EHRs in small practices.

Health Information and Management Systems Society
www.himss.org

The Health Information and Management Systems Society (HIMSS) is a membership organization that promotes optimal use of health information technology and management systems to improve human health. With more than 15,000 individual and 200 corporate members, HIMSS aims to lead health care policy and industry practices through advocacy, education, and professional development initiatives.

> ### EHR Tracking Issues for HIMSS
>
> ▶ Davies recognition of exemplary EHR implementations
>
> ▶ Collaborative activities
>
> ▶ Integrating Healthcare Enterprise (IHE)
>
> ▶ Annual conference trade show

One such initiative is the Nicholas E. Davies EHR Recognition Program that promotes excellence in EHR system implementation and recognizes provider organizations successfully using EHR systems to improve health care delivery. This program demonstrates the vision of EHR via concrete examples, documents the value of EHR systems, and showcases high-impact systems and successful implementation. Another program co-sponsored by HIMSS is the Integrating the Healthcare Enterprise (IHE) initiative, started in 1998 to create the framework for seamlessly passing health information via computer systems across all units of the health care enterprise.

For medical practices seeking EHR solutions, the HIMSS annual conference presents a large trade show for health information technology products and services, typically featuring more than 600 exhibitors.

Integrated Health Association
www.iha.org

```
001010010110100101001010100
```

EHR Tracking Issues for IHA

▶ Pay-for-performance measures and results

▶ Public reporting measures

▶ Testing measures

▶ e-prescribing

Some health plans have indicated that they are willing to pay for performance (P4P) based on the use of an EHR. An example is the Integrated Health Association (IHA), an umbrella agency for six California P4P bonus programs initiated in 2003. The participating health insurance companies are Aetna, Blue Cross of California, Blue Shield of California, CIGNA HealthNet, and PacifiCare. The Pacific Business Group on Health (PBGH) sets standards upon which IHA measures performance. Examples of these measures include chronic care indicators, preventive screenings, and immunizations. Many of the performance measures are based on drug use guidelines, which can be supported by EHR and e-prescribing. In addition, IHA considers patient satisfaction and investment in IT infrastructure. IHA and PBGH work together to collect data and jointly publicize performance scores, which they publish. Each member of IHA has its own incentive payment distribution formula based on common performance measures.

Institute of Medicine
www.iom.edu

```
001010010110100101001010100
```

EHR Tracking Issues for IOM

▶ Quality indicators

▶ Patient safety recommendations

▶ Key capabilities of EHRs

▶ Inventory of organizations working to create a more patient-responsive health system

The Institute of Medicine (IOM) is an independent, non-profit organization that is part of the National Academies. It is organized to provide science-based advice on biomedical science, medicine and health. IOM has published a number of well-read and widely referenced reports based on an ongoing effort focused on assessing and improving the quality of care in the United States.

The initial phase of the quality initiative, starting in 1996, addressed the serious and pervasive nature of the health care quality problems facing the nation. The second phase, from 1999 to 2001, constructed a vision on how to transform the health care system and health care policy development process to close the chasm between what is known to be good quality care and the care that is being delivered. The second phase reports include:

- ▶ To Err is Human: Building a Safer Health System; and

- ▶ Crossing the Quality Chasm: A New Health System for the 21st Century

A discussion of *Crossing the Quality Chasm: The IOM Health Care Quality Initiative*, including the reports for the quality initiative, can be found at www.iom.edu (choose Reports, and search for "Quality Chasm"). Many of the patient safety and quality issues raised can be improved through the use of EHRs. The Quality Chasm reports discuss how to use quality indicators and patient safety improvements in EHRs, and they list several organizations working to support a more patient-responsive health system in the 21st century.

Workgroup for Electronic Data Interchange
www.wedi.org

The Workgroup for Electronic Data Interchange (WEDI) is a non-profit trade association focused on electronic connectivity in the health care industry. WEDI has played a leading industry role in the implementation of HIPAA and has expanded its role to include the electronic connectivity of clinical information. Monitor the WEDI Web site regularly to stay informed of new events, resources and legislative news regarding EHRs.

WEDI is conducting a pilot study of the implementations of the electronic claims attachment, which will be used to demonstrate the feasibility

> **EHR Tracking Issues for WEDI**
>
> - ▶ Business/clinical interoperability
> - ▶ e-prescribing
> - ▶ Regional collaborations focused on data interchange
> - ▶ Security and privacy white papers
> - ▶ EHR implementation
> - ▶ Electronic claims attachment pilot project

and best practices of implementing that HIPAA transaction, including the acquisition and communication of the electronic clinical information for the attachments. WEDI's workgroups have developed white papers and conducted policy advisory group programs to build consensus across the health care industry on the issues of communicating information electronically. More than 30 WEDI white papers exist on HIPAA privacy, security, and transactions. In 2004, WEDI was named by CMS to provide advice on the pilot test of the claims attachment transaction.

▶ Conclusion

The sample of government entities, standards development organizations, and associations presented here will keep you informed of ongoing legislation, recommendations, and decisions regarding EHRs. But they are not the only resources available. Their Web sites will guide you to other sources of information, including other Web sites. It will benefit you and your practice to take advantage of these resources.

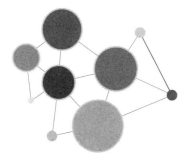

► TEN

EHR Case Study

The following EHR case study is based on representative experiences of several medical groups as they have gone through the process of developing a strategic plan, selecting and implementing an EHR, and monitoring ongoing operations.

THIS CASE STUDY HIGHLIGHTS the type of issues and decisions medical groups face when selecting and implementing an EHR. This is a far more involved process than the information technology (IT) used by the vendor and the IT infrastructure for your medical group. If you decide to implement an EHR with more capability than just recording and retrieving paper record images, this case study will help you:

► Address the significant consideration that must be given to understanding and supporting the best business and clinical practice work flow for your organization's training and utilization issues;

> ### The Case Study Environment
>
> The Do It Right Medical Group is a single-specialty group practice of 15 practitioners in multiple locations within a 100-mile radius. The primary facility has a full range of diagnostic testing and procedure capabilities, such as that typically found in hospitals and some mid-size to larger medical groups.

▶ Appreciate the significant components of physician leadership support and visionary staff;

▶ Define the internal practice goals and maintain focus on them; and

▶ Utilize the information given by this case study for other purposes.

▶ Determining the Requirements and Strategic Plan

The Do It Right Medical Group is fortunate to have as part of its internal resources a visionary chief operations officer (COO), Chris Meadows, who functions as the clinic operations manager. Chris has a good working relationship with the physicians and administrative staff, and was assigned the leadership role to plan the EHR project.

Chris organized an EHR team consisting of the finance director, the IT director, and a physician assistant. Two physicians were identified as sponsors of the project; although these physicians did not regularly attend EHR team meetings, Chris frequently reported to them on the team's progress. The sponsor physicians, together with the COO, were able to effectively tap into the physician leadership for input and guidance on a timely basis.

Requirements

In conducting its requirements analysis, the EHR team reviewed the capabilities of the group's practice management system and identified the key requirements from the clinicians' perspectives. This was done through EHR requirements interviews as well as through scenario construction, in which the EHR team (primarily Chris and the physician assistant) constructed work flow scenarios to describe how the clinicians currently practice and how they could practice with the EHR. The scenario construction and review, together with the probing interviews, led to the following key elements:

▶ Work flow improvement was a key requirement for the EHR. The specialists already worked in a similar manner, so they understood the attractiveness of practicing the same way with regard to work flow and the utilization of evidence-based best-practice templates. Productivity and quality of care were the driving metrics for this objective.

▶ To support the work flow of the physicians and other clinicians, the EHR had to be mobile, so wireless communication became a system requirement.

▶ The EHR had to be fast, which eventually drove the group to seek EHR solutions that operated rapidly in a wireless environment. This has more to do with the EHR software applications design than with wireless performance.

▶ The physicians were used to dictating, and they did it very rapidly. Even though they desired dictation as an option where absolutely needed (e.g., for exceptional situations for specific patient documentation for which predefined pull-down descriptions are not appropriate), the work flow scenarios led the physicians to understand that they needed to record the data digitally while they were with the patient so that it could be incorporated into the work flow logic structure of the EHR. The physicians expressed a preference for using "point-and-click" instead of keyboard approaches.

▶ Scheduling of not only the patient to see the physician but also all of the procedures and treatments, as well as the personnel and rooms for them, had to be integrated with the EHR work flow. This requirement led the practice to prioritize EHRs with a strong, fully integrated scheduling system, rather than to rely on a scheduling system within the PMS.

▶ Due diligence review by the EHR team members revealed that physicians were not always documenting everything they did, which was impacting their diagnosis and procedure coding. This resulted in a requirement that the EHR provide capability for coding and diagnosis review while the physician or physician's assistant records the patient care activity.

▶ Lost charges were found to be a problem, particularly for hospital visits and work that was performed in some of the satellite locations. The EHR requirements therefore included a capability to deploy the EHR enterprise-wide and to extend it into the hospital. (It was understood at the time that deployment to the hospital might be a future activity that was not part of the initial implementation, but the group members wanted to assure that they could move in this direction as soon as they were able and the hospitals permitted it.)

Strategic Plan

Based on the findings of the requirements analysis, the group decided that its key strategic goals could be met with an EHR that contained the following characteristics (included in the requirements analysis):

▶ The EHR had to employ mobile, wireless handheld devices with a display area big enough for clinicians to be able to read and document data, based on point-and-click data entry and retrieval.

▶ Data accessibility had to be rapid, with minimal delay in the work flow of the clinicians.

▶ The system had to have full interoperability and the ability to be deployed enterprise-wide in multiple locations.

▶ The work flow and screens had to be intuitively obvious to the clinicians to minimize training time and to support needed functionality.

▶ The EHR had to have a robust scheduling system that was fully integrated with the work flow.

▶ Clinical decision support and work flow management of clinical results (e.g., labs) had to be fully integrated into the EHR work flow capability.

▶ Examples of this EHR product had to be already installed in a comparable group of this size, or convincingly scalable to this size of organization (i.e., more than 40 EHR users, comparable to the size of the group's 15 practitioners plus their support staff).

▶ Clinician coding for billing had to be supported, and there had to be an automated flow from documented activity to billing application.

▶ e-prescribing by fax (a requirement) had to include the ability to create and store individual patient pharmacy/fax number lists. The system had to have the capability to permit the physicians to move to e-prescribing via electronic data interchange (EDI) consistent with Medicare requirements.

▶ Pre-Selection Phase

The physician EHR sponsors reviewed and approved the criteria for moving forward to the system selection phase. At this stage, it was understood that there might be a need to change the current PMS due to potential difficulties in establishing workable bi-directional interfaces between the EHR and the existing PMS. It was also understood that the PMS vendor was working on an EHR proposal, but the demonstrations seen to date were far from being responsive to the group's requirements.

The EHR team created a return on investment (ROI) model based on the estimated cost for the EHR and hardware, support, and the benefits that it expected to achieve, especially with regard to increased revenue from lost charges and proper coding, as well as from increased productivity. The results looked favorable, with a positive ROI in less than three years. The finance director confirmed that access to capital was not a major barrier if the numbers remained attractive. The group had a good track record with its bank, so it would have no problem borrowing the required capital at attractive rates.

A final, but important, step taken in moving forward to the selection stage occurred at the next scheduled quarterly physician practice retreat. A physician leader from a group practice in the same specialty from another state was invited to speak to all of the physicians on the work flow, cultural, and medical practice changes that occurred in his organization when it implemented an EHR. For this meeting, the physician assistants and the members of the EHR team were invited as observers – something that had never occurred before in this medical group. The presenting physician provided a credible source of realistic expectations for all of the physicians, and gave leadership several insights as to the important change aspects they would have to address to be successful. During the discussion at the physician retreat, one physician questioned how all of this could be accomplished successfully. She had taken the time to visit a group practice in the community that had tried to implement an EHR and had failed. In fact, that group had the same PMS as the Do It Right Medical Group. After spending several hundred thousand dollars and more than a year of effort, the other group in the community had decided to abandon the EHR project. Before Chris, the COO of the Do It Right Medical Group, could respond, one of the two physician sponsors made the following key points:

▶ Based on information available to date, the Do It Right Medical Group EHR team realized that the EHR offered by the practice's PMS vendor was not adequate to meet the group's needs;

▶ A brief review of the highlights of the EHR criteria being pursued was presented; and

▶ The physician also indicated the plan to hire an EHR consultant and add support to the IT infrastructure to minimize risk of failure in the selection and implementation process.

The underlying message delivered by the sponsoring physician was that the Do It Right Medical Group was aware that certain risks are involved in an EHR project and that leadership was prepared to invest in minimizing the risk of failure and maximizing the ROI for the group and its patients. Having a physician leader express this preparation and awareness had a positive impact on the "doubting" physicians in the group, although it did not totally relieve their concerns.

This exchange among the physicians provided an increased level of confidence in the EHR team that it could be successful because the physician sponsor understood the issues and was able to communicate them in a positive way to his colleagues. It was at that point the EHR team members knew that they were not acting on their own but had very strong support from their physician sponsors and others.

▶ EHR Selection Process

It was at this point that the EHR team, together with the practice's board of directors, engaged a highly reputable consulting firm to reduce the risk of making the wrong decision on the EHR vendor and/or the PMS vendor's capability to interface to the desired requirements. The consultant had documented EHR experience, as well as expertise with PMS software and how adoption of an EHR would impact work flow in a medical group. So at this time the EHR team added a consultant and hired an IT staff expert in networks, personal computers (PCs), and user interfaces. In addition, the physician assistant and COO (who was essentially the chief information officer as well at this point) were assigned three-quarter-time responsibility to the team to work through the selection and implementation process. Most of the clinic operations responsibilities of the COO were taken over by another individual in the practice, and the practice hired an additional physician assistant for clinical work. This was a significant investment in staffing and consulting for the group, but the physicians understood that their clinical practice would change in many dramatic ways if they were successful, and they needed to invest to assure achieving success.

Through the consultant's understanding of the EHR vendor product landscape and the requirements developed by the medical group, a short list of EHR vendors was constructed based on the EHR vendor capabilities available at the time of the selection.

The group found an EHR vendor solution that met its criteria and allowed the practice to customize the decision support and screen flows to accommodate its needs. That was the good news. In this process, the EHR team members realized that it was unlikely they would be successful in creating appropriate interfaces with the existing PMS that would work to support registration, data transfer, and billing. The barrier was the legacy PMS vendor and its reluctance to cooperate to support this interface.

Even though the group originally was not interested in changing PMS vendors, this barrier caused the practice to examine the PMS offering of the EHR vendor that it had selected. The group found that it was fully integrated with the EHR, adequate for its business needs, and offered at an attractive price when licensed in conjunction with the EHR. This avoided the cost of programming interfaces to the PMS. Therefore, the unplanned-for decision was made to select and implement the EHR and PMS from the same vendor.

▶ The Negotiation

The negotiation between the physician group and the vendor largely focused on three issues:

- ▶ Placing the source code of the current and upgraded versions of the EHR and PMS software applications in escrow in case the vendor went out of business or stopped maintaining and upgrading the application;
- ▶ Determining a staged payment schedule based on milestones; and
- ▶ Creating a license fee schedule that was attractive to the practice for any additional user licenses needed over the next four years.

The parties readily agreed to the first two issues. The medical practice desired a discounted license fee schedule for additional users for an extended period of time because it had plans to expand and did not want the cost of adding users to the EHR to be a major barrier to the expansion plans. After much discussion, and to close the sale, the vendor eventually agreed to hold a favorable expanded license fee structure in place for several years. There was some discussion around issues related to the initial pricing, but this was a minor point to the medical group because the proposed license fee structure was reasonable compared to the marketplace, and the group was allowed to buy its own hardware directly at the best prices it could find, as long as the hardware met the vendor specifications. The EHR vendor was included as a candidate in the hardware selection process.

Two important terms were negotiated: (1) to mitigate the cost of implementation failure and (2) to assure the ability to continue to use the EHR software if the vendor went out of business. The first of these was accomplished by developing a staged payment schedule based on milestones. The milestones used by the Do It Right Medical Group were:

- ▶ Signed contract;

- ▶ Delivery, installation, and initial operational testing of servers with the applications;

- ▶ Successful test of transferring data bi-directionally between the EHR and PMS per the specifications in the request for proposal;

- ▶ First productive use of the PMS;

- ▶ First productive use for 30 days of the EHR in one location by one or more physicians; and

- ▶ First productive use of the EHR in three or more locations or first productive use of the EHR in one location plus 90 days, whichever occurs first.

In regard to the last milestone, certain detailed provisions for the 90 days of use included the ability to utilize all reports with live data (to the extent live data were available) without error by the end of 90 days. Errors or problems identified during that period were to be corrected to the practice's satisfaction within 10 business days for this milestone to be measured. For those errors that could not be corrected within 10 business days, the milestone definition was changed to 90 days after the last error correction.

The second protection for the medical group was the requirement to place the current and future and every upgraded version of the EHR and PMS software applications in escrow with a third party. In placing the source code in escrow, the medical group was assured that if the vendor company went into bankruptcy, or if "fatal" errors or bugs occurred that were not corrected within 60 days, the group would have access to the source code for its own ongoing use and would be allowed on its own to modify the source code as needed. As part of this protection, the medical group had the right to inspect the source code periodically to make sure it reflected the current version of each application. This provision gave the group protection if the vendor went bankrupt, failed to fix significant problems with the software applications, or discontinued upgrades to the product to the point where it would not meet regulatory requirements. Should any of these shortfalls occur, the medical group had the right to access and use the source code with its own or contacted programmers to maintain the system. Although this alternative might be costly, at least the group would have the option of evaluating it instead of being stuck with a system that isn't being upgraded to meet regulations or having to buy a new system to replace the EHR and PMS.

Once these negotiations were ironed out, the administrator, the COO, and one of the physician sponsors presented an EHR plan and requirements to the clinical and non-clinical staff at a regular staff meeting. This set the initial stage for preparing the entire staff for the change that would occur and alerted clinical and non-clinical staff to the need for their participation in the EHR customization and other aspects of the project. Staff then were updated on a quarterly basis on project progress until implementation began, at which time the staff updates occurred monthly.

▶ Paper Chart Conversion

The medical group decided not to scan all of the paper charts as the means to convert them. This decision was made due to the large volume of charts, the generally large size of each chart, and the inability to utilize the data for decision support if it were scanned.

Instead, the group took an approach that involved abstracting key information from each chart onto a template, and then selecting specific reports in the chart for scanning. The rest of the chart would then be archived for at least six years off site.

The first approach to this process was tried with medical records staff and nurses. The abstracting part worked well, but the selection of key documents to be scanned did not. In a second approach, the medical records staff and nurses prepared the abstract prior to each established patient being seen the first time after implementation. The electronic abstract was in the EHR, and the physician viewed it while also having access to the paper chart. During the patient visit, the physician reviewed the chart and indicated which of the documents in the chart should be scanned into the EHR. This process worked well and provided a quality conversion.

▶ Implementing the EHR and PMS

Productivity Goals

Three key steps were taken to minimize the risk to the implementation to assure that the productivity goals were met.

First, the medical group customized the screen presentations and work flow decision support to the scenarios desired for the group. These were then tested by two physicians for 100 patients each. The patients were a combination of new patients and follow-up patients. After the completion of the pilot, EHR use was discontinued while the EHR team and the physicians reviewed their findings. Based on the experience of the pilot, they decided to totally reconstruct the decision support, work flow, and screens to reflect and improve the process to one that was more intuitive to the physicians. This was a key step in physician acceptance and minimizing training issues, especially for physicians.

Second, during the pilot, each of the patients who were treated when the physician utilized the EHR was handed a short questionnaire about the experience. Because the patient mix of this practice included a significant number of Medicare recipients, there was some concern about the potential reaction of patients to the use of an electronic notepad in the examining room. The analysis of the survey data revealed that almost all of the patients were either neutral or very pleased with the use of the computer. Many noted that they felt more confident of the physician because the physician was utilizing a computerized tool as part of the process. This finding resolved concerns the practice had about negative impacts of the EHR on patients. In part, these findings may reflect the use of a mobile notepad that the physician placed on the side of the table while facing the patient, much like the previous use of the paper chart to make notes while interviewing the patient.

Third, the practice offered two types of training for all clinicians. There was group in-person training for two to four hours held on the evenings and on Saturdays at each location just before going live. During the first two weeks of implementation at each site, two members of the EHR team – a technical IT person and a physician assistant trainer – were present to answer questions and provide support on an ongoing basis on site.

Method of Implementation

The group did decide to implement the EHR site by site, with the main campus going first. Once the internal implementation was completed, the organization began working on data feeds into the EHR. One of the first ones tackled was the data feed from the major external laboratory. The group also developed data feeds from some of the diagnostic devices directly into the EHR. It found that work flow improved significantly, increasing its capacity to see more patients and perform more tests within the same period of time each day. Additional ROI occurred by capturing the previously lost charges from the satellite practices. Initially, the hospitals would not allow the use of the wireless devices inside their facilities, so the medical group, in collaboration with the vendor, developed a stand-alone EHR version that could be used in the hospital to capture information about the patients being seen there for billing and other purposes. This helped with charge capture and treatment planning for the hospitalized patients. At the time of implementation, the practice added a database administrator to support the multiple reporting needs, including clinical research.

HIPAA Privacy and Security Rules

The medical group used the EHR and PMS implementation as an opportunity to review its Health Insurance Portability and Accountability Act of 1996 (HIPAA) privacy and security policies and procedures, and to revisit its HIPAA security risk analysis. This review revealed many new opportunities with the PMS and EHR applications to improve the organization's performance on privacy and security by utilizing the technical functional support available in these new applications. For example, audit trails could automatically be created, stored, and analyzed with the new applications, whereas the legacy PMS did not have this capability except to track the last person who altered a patient data field. Role-based access became easier to administer, and the training program for the EHR and PMS emphasized the need for each individual to utilize his/her own identifier and password, not only for compliance with HIPAA security but also to correctly identify in the EHR who was placing orders, responding to telephone calls, and signing the patient chart. All of these functions are linked directly to the individual's sign-on and authentication in the EHR and PMS. These new capabilities resulted in some of the HIPAA privacy and security policies and procedures being revised; appropriate revisions were also made to HIPAA privacy and security training.

Problem Resolution

The medical group did have to address one problem with the vendor early in the implementation. The first trainer that the vendor sent to train the medical group's trainers lacked good communication skills and did not understand the vendor product very well. After two days of on-site work with this individual, the COO called the vendor and requested that the trainer be replaced and the training be rescheduled in a week or two. Reluctantly, the vendor agreed to this request, sending a new, much more experienced trainer two weeks later, and the vendor agreed to waive the fees for the training provided by the first trainer.

For the most part, all of the technical aspects of the EHR implementation went well. The wireless devices worked well and, despite concern that the access points would become overloaded with wireless users, the network was not challenged by too many users trying to access the network through the several access points used in the main facility.

▶ Post-Implementation Issues

Merger Considerations

About six months after the implementation was completed, the Do It Right Medical Group entered into negotiations with a smaller group of physicians in the same specialty to merge the practices. One of the assets that the Do It Right Medical Group bought to the merger was the EHR and the benefits that could be achieved through improved work flow, productivity, changes for revenue capture, and overall patient and provider satisfaction. However, the other group wanted to keep control of the financial aspects of its practice by maintaining its own billing office and continuing to use its existing PMS. With very little discussion, the physician leaders of the Do It Right Medical Group refused to proceed with any further discussion because they understood that one of the keys to the future success of the merger included a common infrastructure for everyone that included the billing system. The physicians' concerns also included their belief in the importance of integrating the other practice's appointment scheduling system with EHR, and that a costly and resource-intense project would occur if they tried to interface the other practice's legacy PMS to their existing applications. It turned out that this was a deal breaker, and the merger did not occur. The Do It Right Medical Group went on to find other merger opportunities and grew the practice. The group remains consistent with its vision for business operations to provide quality of care to patients in an enterprise-wide environment that supports access to electronic data and decision support.

Cost Savings

As part of its post-implementation plan, the Do It Right Medical Group identified that several of its payers offered pay-for-performance (P4P) incentives tied to measurable quality improvements in a number of clinical areas. The group's new EHR facilitated the rapid and accurate capture of these data, and the practice was able to defray some of its operating expenses through increased payments. In addition, the group began to explore the possibility of decreased malpractice insurance premiums, noting that several local carriers offered discounts when physicians utilized EHR and e-prescribing. The practice also systematically continually monitored federal government and industry Web sites for news on the adoption of new standards that would impact the organization and the development of additional P4P programs. (See Chapter 9, The Regulatory and Standards Environment, for examples of such sources.)

Server Capacity

About a year after full implementation, the server supporting the EHR and PMS data began to fill up. The EHR team, in its budget preparation and planning for a multi-year budget, indicated to the board of directors that additional server capacity would be required as the database grew. In the following budget year, the medical group ignored this warning and decided not to expand server capacity. As the server capacity exceeded 90 percent, the system response time slowed, but the group put off increasing the server capacity. One day, the server just shut down because there was no capacity left to store the data. It took two days to acquire and install additional server capacity and bring the system back up to full use again. During those two days, no patient records were accessible with full EHR functionality. This was a lesson well learned that probably will never happen again in this organization.

Data Retrieval

When a pharmaceutical manufacturer announced a drug recall for a medication that had been widely prescribed by the medical group, within one hour, all of the patients who had been prescribed this medication were identified. Those who did not have a scheduled appointment within the next week received a phone call that day to bring them in to the practice to meet with their physicians to discuss changing medication, and the patients were instructed as to whether they should continue use of their existing supply or stop using the medication until they talked with their physicians. If the practice had been utilizing paper charts, this would have been an impossible task. The physicians would have no choice but to wait for patients who were taking the drug to call in to determine what they should do. Instead, the practice could be proactive, providing timely support to its patients for changing medications.

▶ Conclusion

This case study is presented for educational purposes. Although it does not cover all aspects of EHR planning and implementation, it does illustrate examples of decisions and actions that were made during the process, which could have significance in your own decision making as you implement and sustain an EHR for your practice.

24x7 – Referring to computer availability 24 hours a day, 7 days a week; never shutting down.

A

Acceptance testing – A test of how well the computer system works after being implemented and before making a final payment or accepting the product as final.

Access – The ability of a user or computer system to view, change, or communicate with an object in a computer system.

Access control – The prevention of unauthorized use of a resource. In health care, access control is often designated as user based (access dependent only on who is accessing data), role based (access based not only on who is doing the accessing, but also on the role of that individual at the time of access, such as attending physician or consultant), or context based (access controlled based on who is doing the accessing, what role that person has, and what specific data elements that person has authority to access).

Accredited Standards Committee (ASC) X12N – The standards development organization that has developed standards for financial and administrative transactions, such as 837 – Health Care Claim, 835 – Health Care Claim payment/Advice, and others. This sometimes is called ANSI X12, which is incorrect because the American National Standards Institute (ANSI) accredits standards committees but does not create standards.

Accuracy – Errors in data resulting from miscoding or misrepresenting facts, maintaining out-of-date findings, or co-mingling of data from more than one person.

Adverse drug event (ADE) – The harmful result of a medication, whether or not it is a result of a medication error.

Agency for Healthcare Research and Quality (AHRQ) – Part of the U.S. Department of Health and Human Services that funds research and demonstration projects relating to health care quality, including the impact of EHR systems on quality.

Aggregate data – Data elements assembled into a logical format to facilitate comparisons or to elicit evidence of patterns. Aggregated health care data often, although not necessarily, contain data that can identify the patient and/or provider, even though the information is removed.

Alert – Health care warnings based on a set of rules that are generated through a computer. Alerts often display on a computer screen. An alarm is a similar type of warning but is often generated from an automated medical device.

Algorithm – A mathematical model used to solve a specific computational problem. Used in clinical decision support systems to compare data against specific rules and provide alerts or reminders.

Application service provider (ASP) – A third-party entity that manages and distributes software-based services and solutions to customers across a wide area network from a central data center. In essence, ASPs are a way for practices to outsource some or almost all aspects of their information technology needs and to manage the financing of EHR acquisition.

ASTM International – A standards development organization that has been in existence for more than one hundred years with its primary focus being on the testing of materials to ensure their consistency. For example, motor oil is graded according to ASTM standards. ASTM E31, a committee within ASTM, creates standards on content, structure, and functionality of EHR systems.

Analog – Of, or related to or being a device based on waveforms rather than on binary patterns of voltage.

Architecture – The configuration, structure, and relationships of hardware in an information system.

Audit trail – The chronological set of records that provides evidence of system activity. Data are collected about every system event (log-ins and log-outs, file accesses) and used to facilitate the determination of security violations.

Authentication – Proof of authorship that ensures, as much as possible, that log-ins and messages from a user originate from an authorized source. Authentication of a user can be done in one of three ways: by something the user knows (password), by something the user has (computer token), or by something the user provides (a written signature or fingerprint).

Authorization – The granting of permission to disclose confidential, protected health information.

B

Backup – The process of ensuring that a copy of all software and data is maintained for use should the primary source become compromised.

Backward compatibility – The capability of a software or hardware product to work with earlier versions of itself.

Bandwidth – The range of frequencies a device or communication medium is capable of carrying.

Batch processing –The collection of computer tasks to run at one time, such as at night.

Benefits – Achievement of results based on changes in work flow and processes as a result of the EHR.

Benefits portfolio – The notion that the benefits (of an EHR) are not just financial. Increasingly, quality, patient safety, productivity, and patient satisfaction are identified as equally important benefits.

Benefits realization – The study of the benefits actually received by implementing a new system.

Biometrics – The physical characteristics of users (such as fingerprints, voiceprints, retinal scans, iris traits) that systems store and use to authenticate identity before allowing the user access to a system.

Break-the-glass – A means of providing access to data in a computer system in which access controls would normally prevent access. In HIPAA, this is called emergency access procedures.

Broadband – Describes communications media that can transmit multiple channels of data simultaneously.

Browser – A program that provides a way to view and read the documents available on the World Wide Web.

Bugs – Idiosyncrasies in software that prevent smooth application function.

Business case – An economic argument, or justification, usually for a capital expenditure such as a CPR system.

C

Capital budget – A plan of proposed outlays for acquiring long-term assets and sources of funds to finance them.

Clinician – In this reference, all professionals (physicians, nurses, technologists, therapists, and others) who provide care directly to patients. Caregivers who are nonprofessionals but take care of relatives, friends, or clients or who are themselves patients and assume the role of caregiver in self-care are distinguished from clinicians who are specially trained professionals.

Care plans – Procedures for performing health care for a specified patient.

Cash flow – Receipts less disbursements; the availability of money to pay the organization's bills (accounts payable [A/P]).

Celebration – The act of acknowledging the efforts people have put into something, such as an EHR implementation and associated changes.

Centers for Medicare and Medicaid Services (CMS) – The agency within the federal government responsible for the Medicare and Medicaid programs. Formerly, Health Care Financing Administration (HCFA).

Certificate Authority (CA) – An independent licensing agency that vouches for a person's identity in encrypted electronic communications. Acting as a type of electronic notary public, a CA verifies and stores a sender's public and private encryption keys (in a digital signature) and issues a digital certificate, or "seal of authenticity," to the recipient.

Change management – The formal process of introducing change, getting it adopted, and diffusing it throughout the practice.

Chart – As a noun, refers to the health record of a patient; as a verb, refers to documenting information about a patient in a health record.

Chart conversion – The process of deciding and implementing the means to get data from paper-based charts into the new EHR, such as by abstraction or scanning. Decisions relate to what charts will be converted and for how long paper charts will be retained and retrieved for patient care.

Classification – A system that arranges like or related clinical entities for easy retrieval.

Client/server – A computer architecture in which multiple clients (computers) that help users capture and view data are connected to other computers (servers) that hold the application software and use it to process data sent to the servers from the clients.

Clinical data repository (CDR) – See Data repository.

Clinical data warehouse (CDW) – See Data warehouse.

Clinical decision support (CDS) – The use of automated rules based on clinical evidence to converge information and provide knowledge to the clinician at the point of care to assist in health care delivery.

Clinical guidelines/protocols – With clinical care plans and clinical pathways, a predetermined method of performing health care for a specific disease or other clinical situation based on clinical evidence that the method provides quality and cost-effective health care; also called treatment guidelines/protocols.

Clinical messaging – The capability of exchanging electronic health information via secure web structures.

Clinical trial – Research study in which the effectiveness of a new drug or treatment protocol that has met the initial set of laboratory requirements for safety is provided to one group in a clinical setting, and the outcomes of that group then are compared with those of a control or comparison group that did not receive the same drug or treatment.

Code – A representation; in computers, instructions written to perform an action. Source code is the set of instructions in the application program that is fed into a compiler that produces files the computer can understand and execute (run). In health care, *code* refers to the representation of terms in a classification and/or vocabulary.

COLD (computer output to laser disk) – A system in which documents (e.g., transcribed notes or summaries, or lab results) are transferred from the system creating the data to a laser disk for storage and subsequent retrieval. It is often combined with document imaging to achieve a more complete electronic collection of documents.

Compliance – Conforming to law or regulation. In health care, compliance has come to specifically refer to not acting fraudulently with respect to, or not abusing, the reimbursement system and, generally, to following regulatory and accrediting standards.

Computer-based patient record (CPR) – A term coined by the Institute of Medicine's Patient Record Study Committee in 1991 and used to describe electronically maintained information about an individual's lifetime health status and health care that resides in a system designed to support users by providing accessibility to complete and accurate data, alerts, reminders, clinical decision support systems, links to medical knowledge, and other aids.

Computerized provider order entry (CPOE) – A system typically deployed in hospitals or large practices wherein the provider directly enters orders for distribution to various operational systems or departments for their action. CPOE systems are most effective when coupled with clinical decision support to ensure complete, accurate, and legible orders.

Confidentiality – The act of limiting disclosure of private matters; maintaining the trust an individual has placed in someone who has been entrusted with private matters. Also, it is the status accorded to data or information indicating that it needs to be protected against theft or improper use and must be disseminated only to others authorized to have it.

Consent – The agreement of an individual for a given action relative to the individual. Consent may be expressed in an oral or written agreement or implied through action that demonstrates consent. *Informed consent* refers to the validity of consent; an informed consent follows a careful explanation of what one is agreeing to.

Consumer – A person buying goods or services. In health care, the consumer may be a patient, client, resident, or other recipient of health care services.

Contextual – Depending upon the parts of a written or spoken statement that precede or follow a specified word or phrase and can influence the meaning or effect of the word or phrase. Because the language of health care is contextual, it is difficult to automate. (For example, "red" may mean hot in the context of "red hot," or a color in the context of "red spot.")

Contingency plan – Preparation made for responding to a system emergency. A contingency plan includes performing backups, preparing critical facilities that can be used to facilitate continuity of operations in the event of an emergency, and recovering from a disaster.

Continuity of care record (CCR) – A content specification developed by the standards organization, ASTM International and several medical specialty societies. Provides a standard set of data for referrals.

Continuum of care – The full range of health care services from lowest to highest intensity.

Controlled vocabulary – Predefined set of terms and their meanings that may be used in structured data entry or natural language processing to represent expressions. Also called standard vocabulary.

Cost/benefit analysis – The comparison of system costs against system benefits to determine the value of the system.

Current Procedural Terminology® (CPT®) – Coding system developed by the American Medical Association for the reporting of procedures and services.

Cryptography – The art of keeping data secret, primarily through the use of mathematical or logical functions that transform intelligible data into seemingly unintelligible data and back again.

D

Data – A sequence of symbols that have limited meaning without context and further processing. A data element is the smallest unit of a fact or value that is stored in a computer. Data are the raw material of information, which is data that have been processed to produce something that was not known before.

Data analyst – An individual who understands the sources and uses of data in a health care environment and is responsible for planning, organizing and monitoring the data dictionary, database(s), and report management for the organization's business and clinical data needs.

Database – A collection of data structured in logical relationships. Flat-file databases allow users to work with only one data table or set of fields at a time, whereas relational and other newer types of databases compensate for this.

Database administrator (DBA) – An individual who knows DBMS software and can maintain a database structure for optimal performance. This includes managing both data files and indexes to data, data dictionaries, and other attributes of a DBMS (known as metadata, or data about data).

Database management system (DBMS) – Computer software that manages a database.

Data center – A department or specially designed location used to house all main computer equipment in a safe and secure manner.

Data comparability – The property that data from different sources have the same meaning, usually accomplished through a common data dictionary, or ideally through the use of a controlled vocabulary.

Data conversion – The task of moving data from one data structure to another, usually from an old system to a new system at the time of a new system installation.

Data dictionary – A set of terms and their meanings within a database.

Data Encryption Standard (DES) – An encryption algorithm adopted as the federal standard for the protection of sensitive unclassified information and used extensively for the protection of commercial data as well.

Data flow analysis – The process of identifying all data sources and uses to ensure that an EHR you acquire can accommodate all of your data requirements.

Data integrity – The property that data have not been altered or destroyed in an unauthorized manner or by unauthorized users; a security principle that keeps information from being modified or otherwise corrupted either maliciously or accidentally.

Data mining – The process used to query and analyze a data warehouse for trends.

Data model – The definitions of fields and records, and their relationships in a database. By understanding the data model, a database administrator can enforce accuracy and integrity constraints.

Data repository – A database with an open structure that is not dedicated to the software of any particular vendor or data supplier, where data from diverse sources are stored so that an integrated, multidisciplinary view of the data can be achieved; also called *central data repository (CDR)*, or *clinical data repository (CDR)* if related specifically to health care data.

Data retrieval – The process of viewing and comprehending data, the study of which helps to improve the human–machine interface. Results retrieval is the computer application of viewing laboratory and other diagnostic study results.

Data set – A group of data elements relevant for a particular use.

Data structure – The form in which data are stored, as in a file, a database, a data repository, and so on.

Data sources – Data that are captured by your information system from any source – the internal user or an external feeder system.

Data uses – The purposes for which data are captured; the manner in which data are used, shared with others, supplied on claims, or contributed to an internal or external database.

Data warehouse – A database of information that is optimized for analysis across a population of data. Data stored in the warehouse are specially classified and labeled for appropriate use. The warehouse is designed to identify trends and support creation of knowledge, not for day-to-day transactions.

Default – The status to which a computer application reverts in the absence of alternative instructions.

DICOM (Digital Imaging and Communications in Medicine) – Standard protocol for exchanging medical images among computer systems.

Digital – A data transmission type based on data that have been binary encoded.

Digital signature – A means to guarantee the authenticity of a set of input data in the same way that a written signature verifies the authenticity of a paper document; a cryptographic transformation of data that allows a recipient of the data to prove their source and integrity and protect against forgery.

Digital versatile disc (DVD) – A type of generation of compact disc (CD) that can store up to 14 times more data than a CD, making DVDs ideal for multimedia. DVDs and CDs use a laser substance to store data, in comparison to older media that are magnetic, such as floppy disks.

Discipline – The process of adopting and accepting change and following organizational policies and rules where such behavior provides benefits to the whole.

Disclosure – The act of making information known; the release of confidential health information about one person to another person. Disclosure does not imply authorization or lack of authorization.

Discrete data – Data that may be represented individually and that are more concise and processable than imaged data.

Disk mirroring – The creation of an exact copy of one disk from another, for backup.

Documentation – The recording of pertinent health care findings, interventions, and response to treatment as a business record and form of communication among caregivers.

Document imaging – A system of scanning written or printed paper into a computer for later retrieval of the document or parts of the document if parts have been indexed. If optical character recognition (OCR) is used, individual characters can be processed, such as through word processing.

Due diligence – The actions associated with making a good decision, including investigation of legal, technical, human, and financial predictions and ramifications of proposed endeavors with another party.

Durability – The property that media on which data are stored will last for a required period of time.

E

Electronic data interchange (EDI) – The transfer of data between different "trading partners" using network transaction standards from the ANSI Accredited Standards Committee (ASC) X12.

Electronic health record (EHR) – A system that provides for the capture of data from multiple sources and is used as the primary source of information to support clinical decision making at the point of care.

Electronic medical record (EMR) – A term that is often used in physician practices to refer to EHRs. In hospitals, EMR often refers to a document imaging system.

Electronic prescribing (e-prescribing) – A system that supports the creation and transmission of complete, accurate, and legible prescriptions and associated transactions (e.g., refill requests and approvals) between a provider and a pharmacy.

Electronic signature – Any representation of a signature in digital form, including an image of a handwritten signature. It is not as secure as a digital signature.

E/M coding – Evaluation and management coding contained in *Current Procedural Terminology, Edition 4* (*CPT-4*), developed by the American Medical Association and used for documenting physician services for billing purposes. The codes, which represent the level of service performed by the physician, have been developed into application programs that can be used to prompt physicians for documentation to support the level of service rendered.

Encoder – A computer program that helps assign diagnostic or procedural codes according to the rules of the coding system. The term *encoder* has a broader meaning in computer science, meaning the assignment of symbols (codes) to any set of data.

Encryption – The process of transforming text into an unintelligible string of characters that can be transmitted over communications media with a high degree of security and then decrypted when it reaches a secure destination. See also cryptography.

Evaluation and Management (E&M) – CPT codes that describe the nature of the presenting problem and the skill, effort, time, responsibility and medical knowledge required for the prevention or diagnosis and treatment of illness or injury.

Evidence-based medicine – The term often used to describe clinical decision support, reflecting the notion that such support is based on evidence of best practices rather than an arbitrary set of rules.

Expert system – The term may be used to describe artificial intelligence in medicine, in which a highly sophisticated computer system makes a decision to take action independent of the cognitive intention of the human user. It also may be used to describe any system that provides knowledge for decision making.

Explanation of benefits (EOB) – Also called remittance advice, this is information returned to a provider describing the payments a health plan will make based on a patient's benefits.

F

Feeder systems – Information systems that operate independently of an EHR system but provide data to it; also called source systems. An example of a feeder system includes a laboratory information system.

Firewall – A computer that controls access to an Internet-connected network.

Fixed cost – A cost that does not vary with the number of units of the item being purchased, in contrast to variable cost, in which the cost varies per unit.

Flat-panel display – Technology using a liquid crystal display (LCD) or other low-emission substances, once found primarily on laptops and now being used for desktop monitors, large-screen wall monitors, and HDTV.

Formulary – List of drugs that a pharmacy stocks; under pharmacy benefits management (PBM) programs, the drugs that are covered under a health plan.

FTP (file transfer protocol) – Communications protocol that enables users to copy files among computers.

Full redundancy – A computer architecture in which there are two complete sets of servers and their software which store data. This is a contingency measure in the event that data become corrupted or lost or servers are rendered inoperable for any reason.

Full-time equivalents (FTE) – A numeric statement of the number of people in an organization if all worked a standard work week. For example, if there are three people, but one works full time and two work half time, the number of FTEs is 2.0. FTEs are often used in return on investment (ROI) analysis by vendors to produce positive results, even though partial employees cannot be released.

Functional requirements – A statement of the processes a computer system should perform to derive the technical specifications, or desired behavior, of a system.

G

Gateway – A network that serves as an entrance to another network, such as from a local area network in a practice to the Internet.

"Go Live" – The act of turning over activities to the new system.

Granularity – An expression of the relative size of a unit; the smallest discrete information that can be directly retrieved. Highly granular data are more detailed than non-granular data.

Graphical user interface (GUI) – A style of screen interaction with a computer in which typed commands are replaced by manipulations of pictures (icons), buttons, and menus via a navigational device.

H

Hacker – A person highly skilled in using computers; often used to describe someone who makes unauthorized accesses into others' computer systems, usually maliciously.

Hard-coded – Referring to the fact that a screen displays certain content in accordance with software instructions that cannot be manipulated by the user for purposes of changing the content.

Hardware – Computer and network equipment. Devices used to capture, process, present, transmit, and store data in electronic form.

Hardwire – The use of cable or telephone wires to connect devices within a network, or connect one network to another. See also Wireless.

Health data analyst (HDA) – A person who has a combination of some of the following responsibilities: maintains the integrity and availability of the EHR data dictionary and clinical data repository; trains end-users in report writing and use of standardized reports from the EHR; creates customized reports from the EHR, including those used for research; and creates and uses databases consisting of a subset of the clinical data repository information set for customized studies or submission to others (e.g., public health).

Health information technology – The concept of using information technology (in all forms, including the EHR) in health care to achieve quality, cost, efficiency, and effectiveness benefits.

Health information management (HIM) professional – Individual who has received professional training in the management of health data and flow of information throughout the health care delivery system.

Health information technology (HIT) – The concept of using information technology (in all forms, including the EHR) in health care to achieve quality, cost, efficiency, and effectiveness benefits.

Health Insurance Portability and Accountability Act of 1996 (HIPAA) – Law passed by Congress in 1996 to provide continuous insurance coverage and reduce insurance fraud and abuse. The Administrative Simplification section requires adoption of standards for claims and other financial and administrative transactions, code sets, identifiers, privacy, and security.

Health Level Seven® (HL7®) – An organization created in the 1980s to develop standards for computer systems to share data.

Health plan – An entity that provides or pays the cost of medical care, including a group health plan, a health insurance issuer, a health maintenance organization, or any welfare benefit plan such as Medicare, Medicaid, CHAMPUS, and Indian Health Services. Often also called "payer."

HEDIS (Health Plan Employer Data and Information Set) – A group of performance measures that assesses the results that health plans actually achieve; developed by the National Committee for Quality Assurance (NCQA), which provides an accreditation service for managed care organizations.

Help desk – Central access point to information systems support services that attempts to resolve technical problems, sometimes with the use of decision-making algorithms, and tracks problems until their resolution.

History of present illness (HPI) – Information captured from patients by clinicians to describe the severity, duration, and other aspects of symptoms of illnesses or injuries.

Hospital information system (HIS) – Computer systems within hospitals primarily used to process financial, administrative, and operational data rather than clinical data.

HTML (Hypertext Markup Language) – A standard way of displaying information that allows the user to launch from an icon or word in one document to another document or Web site that has been programmatically linked to it.

HTTP (Hypertext Transport Protocol) – The communications protocol that enables use of linking text from one location to information at another location (often on the Web).

Human-computer interface (HCI) – The device a human uses to enter data on a computer, such as a keyboard, touch screen monitor, speech microphone, personal digital assistant, tablet PC, etc.

I

Informatics – A field of study that focuses on the use of technology for improving access to, and utilization of, information. Health informatics is the broadest view of informatics in health care. Medical and nursing professions also have fields of informatics that focus on those respective domains.

Information technology (IT) – The broad subject concerned with all aspects of managing and processing information using computers and associated tools.

Infrastructure – The underlying framework and features of an information system. Also, in the context of local/regional health information organizations (RHIO) and national health information networks (NHIN) or the national health information infrastructure (NHII), the infrastructure necessary to make exchange of data happen.

Install base – The number of clients for which a vendor has installed a system, as opposed to the number of clients for which a vendor is in the process of selling a system.

Institute of Electrical and Electronic Engineers (IEEE) – The standards development organization that has created standards that support exchange of information with medical devices, certain hardware, and wireless devices (using the standard called IEEE 802.11, of which there are several versions, which may be used for different purposes).

Institute of Medicine (IOM) – A component of the National Academy of Sciences that is a prestigious group composed primarily of physicians who conduct studies and advise Congress on matters pertaining to health care. They have produced a number of reports on patient safety and EHRs.

Integrated Services Digital Network (ISDN) – A network system that transmits voice, data, and signaling digitally and with significantly increased bandwidth compared to traditional T1 lines.

Integration – The complex task of ensuring that all the elements and platforms of an information system communicate and act as a uniform entity. Emerging standards, common languages, interfaces and interface engines (which are computer programs that isolate the task of transferring data from one database to another), and repositories are means of facilitating the integration among information systems.

Integrity – See Data integrity.

Interactive voice response (IVR) – An automated call handler, which can be configured to automatically dial a log of callers and deliver appointment reminders, lab results, and other information when a person answers the phone.

Interface – A program written to enable passage of data between different computer systems.

International Standards Organization (ISO) – Organization that establishes standards in many different areas for many industries so that products and services can be exchanged globally. ISO has established an Open Systems Interconnection (OSI) model for standard worldwide communications.

Internal rate of return (IRR) – A financial analysis of a potential investment, such as in an EHR system, that describes the percent of profit able to be achieved on the investment.

Internet – A worldwide network of interconnected computers to which anyone with a connection may attach and navigate. A portion is called the World Wide Web (WWW), which is a resource that connects large databases and servers to provide electronic mail, education, research, and business.

Internet service provider (ISP) – A company that provides connections to the Internet.

Interoperability – Refers to the capability of systems to work together, passing meaningful information between them.

Intranet – A private Internet network that has its servers located inside a firewall, or security barrier, so that the general public cannot gain access to them.

K

Knowledge management – The process in which data are acquired and transformed into information through the application of context, which in turn provides understanding.

Knowledge sources – Various reference materials and expert information that are compiled in a manner accessible for integration with patient care information (in EHR systems) to improve the quality and cost-effectiveness of health care provision; also called knowledge [data]bases.

L

Leadership – The qualities individuals display in helping a practice adopt new technology, manage change, and implement health information technology.

Learning curve – The pace with which some new information or process can be acquired and comfortably used.

Legacy system – Refers to a computer system that utilizes older technology but may still perform optimally. Legacy systems are affectionately referred to as "systems that work."

Local area network (LAN) – A collection of computers connected to one another in a small area (such as an office or building) in order for users to share programs and devices, such as printers.

Logical Observation Identifiers, Names and Codes® (LOINC®) – A terminology that standardizes laboratory and other terms associated with diagnostic studies for use in clinical care, outcomes management, and research, developed by the Regenstrief Institute for Health Care.

M

Mainframe – A computer architecture built with a single central processing unit (CPU) to which terminals (devices for accessing and entering data without any processing capability) and/or personal computers (PCs, which are then referred to as terminal emulators) are connected. All processing takes place in the CPU, and the terminals serve only to capture and retrieve data. Mainframe systems tend to be considered legacy systems, as they are now being replaced by computers in a client/server architecture or by PCs connected to one another through a network.

Master person index (MPI) – A file of basic demographic data about the patients in a health care organization or the persons enrolled in a managed care organization and the identifiers assigned to those patients or persons to link them with their health records. An enterprise-wide master patient index (EMPI) would integrate all master person indexes in an enterprise so as to achieve a common index in order to identify and, ultimately, to link all the records for a given patient.

Medical record – The compilation of all documentation concerning a person's health care in a given health care organization; also called a *patient record,* a *health record*, or *chart*. A longitudinal (lifetime) health record would be a virtual record or linkage of all health care and health status documentation for a person, regardless of where the documentation took place. Many view a longitudinal (lifetime) health record to be the goal of the EHR.

Medicare Prescription Drug, Improvement, and Modernization Act of 2003 (MMA) – Legislation that provides seniors and people living with disabilities with a prescription drug benefit, more choices of coverage under Medicare, and other reforms intended to control Medicare costs and ensure coverage.

Medication error – A mistake made in the selection, communication, or administration of a medication. A medication error may or may not impact a person's health in a harmful manner, but has the potential to produce a negative outcome. (See also Adverse drug event.)

Migration path – The series of steps required to move from one situation to another. An EHR migration path would describe the systems required to be in place to move from a paper-based health record to an EHR.

Model – A representation of something, such as a process.

Multimedia – The capability of a computer to process data, voice, image, and motion (video) to communicate through a workstation.

N

National Committee for Quality Assurance (NCQA) – Provides accreditation services for managed care organizations.

National Committee on Vital and Health Statistics (NCVHS) – A public advisory body to the U.S. Department of Health and Human Services that recommends data collection standards and provides feedback on health-related regulatory compliance.

National Council for Prescription Drug Programs (NCPDP) – An organization that develops standards for exchanging prescriptions and prescription payment information.

National Health Information Infrastructure (NHII) – A national initiative to improve the effectiveness, efficiency and overall quality of health care in the United States by adopting a comprehensive knowledge-based network of interoperable systems of clinical, public health, and personal health information that would improve decision-making by making health information available when and where it is needed. This is not a centralized database of medical records or a government regulation.

National health information network (NHIN) – A newer term than NHII, which refers to the concept of disparate health care information systems connecting together to allow patients, physicians, hospitals, public health agencies and other authorized users across the nation to share clinical information in real-time under stringent security, privacy and other protections.

National Library of Medicine (NLM) – The world's largest medical library, it is a branch of the National Institutes of Health. Many of its databases are available to the public on the Web. It is the source of the Unified Medical Language System® (UMLS®) designed to help health professionals and researchers retrieve and integrate electronic biomedical information from a number of sources.

National provider identifier (NPI) – Under HIPAA, would replace the Unique Physician Identifier Number (UPIN) for identifying all providers, primarily for billing services under Medicare.

Natural language processing – Automatic extraction of coded medical data from free text. In this way, clinicians do not need to alter the way in which they express their findings or document their decisions, but the individual data elements can be processed.

Net present value (NPV) – A formula used to assess the current value of a project if the monies used were invested in the organization's investment vehicles rather than expended for the project. This value is then compared to the allocation of the monies and the cash inflows of the project, both of which are adjusted to current time.

Networking – The use of specific technology to connect disparate systems so they may share information.

Network capacity management – The process of ensuring that you always have sufficient bandwidth and other network capability to move data among devices on a network. There are several aspects of network capacity management, including the volume, speed, and complexity of data being transmitted.

Network operating system (NOS) – Software that includes special functions for connecting computers and devices into a local-area network (LAN).

O

Online analytical processing (OLAP) – Software tools that can operate on multiple databases to retrieve, analyze, report, and share data from disparate systems, vendors, and departments, such as decision support systems, executive information systems, budgeting, and clinical data repositories.

Online transaction processing (OLTP) – Refers to the real-time processing of day-to-day transactions from a database, such as those used to enter clinical findings into an EHR, retrieve lab results, or receive an alert about a contraindicated medication being prescribed.

Open Systems Interconnection (OSI) – A standard of the International Standards Organization (ISO) for worldwide networking communications that defines a framework for implementing protocols in seven layers.

Operations – The manner of functioning. Typically in a health information technology environment, operational systems are those that help manage financial and administrative functions rather than clinical functions.

Outsourcing – The use of a company separate from the practice to perform work for you. Many computer services can be outsourced, as are billing services, coding services, and others.

P

Password – A sequence of characters an individual provides to a system for purposes of authentication.

Patient portal – A secure entry point from the Internet to a practice's Web page, designed especially for patient use.

Patient safety – The prevention of harm to patients caused by errors of commission and omission in health care.

Payback period – A financial method used to evaluate the value of a capital expenditure by calculating the time frame that must pass before inflow of cash from a project equals or exceeds outflow of cash.

Payer – See Health plan.

Pay for performance (P4P) – A bonus system offered by some payers for medical groups based their results on quality outcomes.

Personal computer (PC) – A computer that designed for an individual user, with full input/output, processing, and storage capability built into the single device.

Personal digital assistant (PDA) – Small computer, often used for personal schedule management and as an address book, although functions have recently been expanded to E/M coding, e-prescribing, and other documentation aids. Many PDAs have wireless connectivity to a practice's network.

Personal health record (PHR) – The maintenance of a health record by a patient, integrating information from various providers and self-reported information. PHRs come in many forms, some electronic (EPHR), others not. Some are originated by a provider, others by the patient.

Pharmacy benefits management (PBM) – Company that manages the complex rules for payers associated with benefit plans to pay for prescription drugs.

Picture archiving and communication system (PACS) – Integrated computer system that obtains, stores, retrieves, and displays digital images; in health care, radiologic images.

Platform – The combination of hardware and operating system on which an application program can run. In reference to platform, an example would be that a PC with a Windows® operating system cannot (easily) run programs designed for an Apple® computer with a Macintosh® operating system. Some application programs run on multiple platforms and thus are cross-platform programs. Other programs must be converted into, or "ported" onto, different platforms in order to run properly.

Point-and-click – A means of data entry in which the user moves the computer's cursor by way of a mouse, up-and-down arrows, or some other pointing, or navigational, device to the desired icon or data element and "clicks" on it to accept it as a link or data.

Point of care – Computer system that captures data at the location (for example, bedside, examination room, or home) where the health care service is performed.

Policy – A statement that describes how an organization is supposed to handle a specific situation.

Practice management system (PMS) – Software that automates a medical practice's patient appointment scheduling, registration, billing, and payroll functions. Many products also provide electronic data interchange (EDI) for filing claims and electronic funds transfer (EFT).

Privacy – Right of an individual to control disclosure of personal information. Under HIPAA, the Privacy Rule sets forth standards for uses and disclosures, patients' rights in, and administrative requirements relative to protected health information

Privilege – A right granted to a user, program, or process that allows access to certain files or data in a system.

Process – Ways people perform work. Computer systems often change processes, ideally for improvement. People often need to manage those change processes to achieve the improvements.

Production environment – The information system processing actual, live data, rather than test data. In comparison, a test environment is a special set of computer equipment used for testing only. In some organizations, both such environments are maintained, so that as upgrades or new systems are installed, the production environment is not disrupted by the testing.

Project manager – The individual designated to help control the activities associated with implementing a usually large undertaking to achieve a specific goal, such as an EHR project. Projects have project executives, managers, plans, sponsors, status reports, teams, timelines, reviews, and vision.

Proprietary – Owned by someone or some organization with rights retained by that person or entity. In computer applications, a system that may not adhere to standard specifications and may not interface well with other systems.

Protected health information (PHI) – The term used in HIPAA to refer to individually identifiable health information to be protected by an entity that must adhere to HIPAA regulations (i.e., a covered entity).

Protocol – An agreed-on standard. In networks, a protocol is used to address and ensure delivery of packets (of data) across a network. In health care, a treatment protocol is a detailed plan of care for a specific health care condition based on investigative studies.

Provider portal – A secure entry point from the Internet to a practice's Web page, designed especially for provider remote access and use of data.

Pull-down menu – Refers to the design of a data-entry screen of a computer in which categories of functions or structured data elements may be accessed through that category element.

Q

Quality of care – The degree of excellence of health care services; meeting expectations for outcomes of care.

R

RAID (redundant array of inexpensive disks) – A form of data storage.

Random access memory (RAM) – Also called "main memory," it is the most common form of internal storage in personal computers, printers, and other electronic devices from which data can be accessed randomly.

Read only memory (ROM) – Special storage component of computers used to store programs that boot the computer (i.e., turn it on) and perform diagnostics.

Real time – Processing performed by a computer system at the time data are entered or requested. Implies interactive use with the computer, in comparison to batch processing.

Record retention – The maintenance and preservation of information in some form.

Regional health information organization (RHIO) – Groups of hospitals, physician practices, and other health-related organizations in a geographic location or region of the country that is interconnected and would collectively form a RHIN.

Reminder – A prompt based on a set of rules that displays on the computer workstation. It is distinguished from an alert or alarm as usually being similar to a recommendation.

Remote access – The capability to access an information system away from the premises, such as from home, via a secure connection through the Internet or direct cable.

Repudiation – A situation in which a user or a system denies having performed some action, such as modifying information. Nonrepudiation services are countermeasures to repudiation in the security environment.

Request for proposal (RFP) – A document in which the practice asks vendors to supply information about their company and products, usually distributed to a small number of vendors for comparison purposes.

Resolution – The degree of sharpness of a computer-generated image as measured by the number of dots per linear inch on a printout or the number of pixels across and down a display screen.

Return on investment (ROI) – The financial analysis of the extent of value a major purchase will provide.

Risk – The aggregate effect of the likely occurrence of a particular threat. In security, a risk assessment may be performed to determine a system's vulnerabilities. A risk analysis may be performed to evaluate the level of security services required to counteract a security threat.

Risk sharing – An agreement in which a vendor assumes at least a part of the responsibility, from a financial perspective, for the successful implementation of a CPR.

Router – A device located at a network's gateway that forwards data along networks. It is connected to at least two networks, such as between two local area networks, or a local area network and an Internet service provider (ISP) network.

Rules engine – A computer program that applies sophisticated mathematical models to data that generate alerts and reminders to support health care decision making.

S

Scalable – The measure of a system to grow. It is not quantifiable but is relative to various measures of size, speed, number of users, volume of data, and so on.

Scanning – The act of using a scanner to capture an image of a document. Scanned documents are part of a document imaging process. Scanned documents may also be used to round out an EHR system where some documents come to the practice only in paper form, not in discrete, or structured, data elements.

Screen layout – the manner in which a data entry format in a computer system is designed for ease of use.

Search engine – A software program used to search for data in databases. An example of such a tool that may be used in an EHR is structured query language (SQL). Search engines are popular tools to find information on the Web (e.g., Google, Yahoo, and many others).

Security (of information) – The means to protect the confidentiality, integrity, and availability of information important to a business. Under HIPAA, the Security Rule provides standards to control access to, audit, and prevent accidental or intentional disclosure, alteration, destruction, or loss of protected health information.

Service level agreement – A part of a contract for services, such as maintenance agreements or outsourced services, that the company contracted with will provide a specified level of service or the contract is subject to being nullified.

Shareware – Software that is freely available from others, often on the Internet, for which a nominal fee is paid. Freeware is similar but is available with no fee whatsoever. Caution should be applied in using shareware or freeware as there may be flaws, minimal documentation, or embedded malicious code.

Single sign-on – Technology that allows a user access to disparate applications through one authentication procedure. Reduces the number and variety of passwords a user must remember when there are multiple different applications; and enforces and centralizes access control.

Smart card – A credit card–sized piece of plastic on which is imbedded a computer chip that may house data and processors for manipulating the data. Smart cards are popular in Europe for maintaining health record data. In the United States, magnetic stripe cards are popular for storing demographic and insurance information, but smart cards have not been widely adopted.

Smart text – A data entry technique that operates much like a word processing macro, using a symbol, word, or set of characters that represents a list of commands, actions, or keystrokes.

Sniffer – A software security product that runs in the background of a network, examining and logging packet traffic and serving as an early warning device against crackers; also called network analyzer or protocol analyzer.

SNOMED CT® (Systematized Nomenclature of Medicine Clinical Terms) – A comprehensive clinical vocabulary developed by the College of American

Pathologists and now freely distributed through SNOMED International under special license from the U.S. National Library of Medicine. It is used in many EHR systems to encode clinical terms for use in clinical decision support systems.

Software – Instructional programs written to work in a computer's processing components to run the equipment (i.e., operating system software) and direct applications (i.e., application software).

Source code – The computer program in which a specific application is written.

Source systems – See Feeder systems.

Speech dictation/recognition – Technology that uses voice patterns to allow computers to record voice and automatically translate it into narrative text in real time. (Voice recognition was an earlier form that required the user to pause between words rather than to use continuous speech.)

Standard – Method, protocol, or terminology agreed on by an industry to allow different systems (often, although not always, from different vendors) to operate successfully with one another.

Standard vocabulary – See Controlled vocabulary.

Standards Development Organization (SDO) – An organization primarily comprised of volunteers from representative concerns who create standards based on due processes described by the American National Standards Institute (ANSI) or International Standards Organization (ISO). For health care, SDOs create standards for interoperability among computer systems and data comparability through controlled vocabularies and standard data sets.

Step list – A means to evaluate work flow, or the steps in a process, usually with the goal of work flow redesign and process improvement through the use of a computer system such as an EHR.

Storage device – A computer device that serves to hold data temporarily or permanently. Some storage devices make data available online in real time. Other storage devices require storage media to be loaded to the device for access (typically used for archiving data).

Structured data entry – The process of capturing data in structured, or discrete, format so that each data element may be processed by a computer. Data elements may be defined in the EHR's data dictionary or, preferably, are defined using a controlled medical vocabulary.

T

TCP/IP (Transmission Control Protocol/Internet Protocol) – The multi-faceted protocol suite, or open standard not owned by or proprietary to any company, on which the Internet runs.

Telemedicine – Telecommunication system that links health care organizations and patients from diverse geographic locations, and transmits text and images for (medical) consultation and treatment.

Template – A pattern, used in EHRs, to capture data in a structured manner.

Terminology – A listing of the proper use of clinical words.

Textual – Referring to the narrative nature of much of clinical documentation to date.

Thick client – A computer with full processing capability and persistent storage.

Thin client – A computer with processing capability (CPU), but no persistent storage (disk memory); relying on data and applications on the server it accesses to be able to process data.

Token – A physical device used to authenticate a computer user.

T1 – A digital phone line that can carry data at speeds of up to 1.544 megabits per second.

Tunneling protocol – A protocol that ensures that data passing over a virtual private network (VPN) are secure; operates as an outer envelope to an enclosure.

Turnkey product – A computer application that may be purchased from a vendor and installed without modification or further development by the user organization.

Turnover – The strategy used to move from the paper-based environment to the computer environment. In general, the turnover options are phased (where certain physicians, locations, or departments are implemented in sequence), parallel (where both paper and electronic are maintained simultaneously), or straight (where there is a specific cutover from paper to electronic for the entire organization).

U

Unified Medical Language System® (UMLS®) – A system of databases and software tools developed by the National Library of Medicine facilitate the development of computer systems that behave as if they "understand" the meaning of the language of biomedicine and health.

Uninterruptible power supply (UPS) – A device that helps power down a computer system safely during a power outage.

Unique Physician Identification Number (UPIN) – An identification number assigned to all physicians who bill Medicare. By 2007, the UPIN will be replaced by the National Provider Identifier which was required by the HIPAA legislation for all health care providers to use with all health plans.

Unstructured data – Data that are captured as a stream of narrative text or an image, rather than as discrete data, each element of which can be processed independently in a computer system.

V

Virtual private network (VPN) – A network established over a carrier's digital phone lines and dedicated solely to connecting several specific client sites.

Virus – A computer program, typically hidden, that attaches itself to other programs and has the ability to replicate and cause various forms of harm to the data. A broader type of harmful program is referred to as malware or malicious software.

Vision – An articulation of the nature and expectations for a future state, especially the long-range plans for achieving a comprehensive EHR and other health information technology. A key element in developing a migration path.

Vocabulary – A list or collection of clinical words or phrases and their meanings. See also Controlled vocabulary.

W

Web-enabled technology – A computer architecture that utilizes World Wide Web technology (for example, browsers that are client software programs designed to look at various kinds of Internet resources) developed for the Internet to connect systems and display data.

Wet signature – Original handwritten signature applied by pen to paper.

Wide area network (WAN) – A series of interconnected local area networks spread across a broad geographical area.

Windows® – An operating system product made by Microsoft®. The system is easy to learn and user-friendly because all applications that run on it have a similar, pictorial appearance and movement among various applications is made available through multiple, simultaneous views.

Wireless – The transmission of data across infrared or radio waves rather than a hardwire cable or telephone line.

Workaround – A series of unnatural steps taken to compensate for either poorly performing software or lack of desire to use a computer.

Work flow – The flow of how processes and functions are performed. As with the processes themselves, EHRs often change work flow for greater efficiency. Work flow is also used specifically as a component of a document imaging system that provides queuing capability to help keep work flowing throughout a practice.

Workstation – A computer that has been designed to accept data from multiple sources to assist in managing information for daily activities and to provide a convenient means of entering data as desired by the user.

World Wide Web (WWW) – See Internet.

X

XML (eXtensible Markup Language) – A system that defines document formats so they may be exchanged by virtually any type of computer applications.

X12 – See Accredited Standards Committee X12N.

Looking for help with additional terms not listed or terms newer than what may be referenced the book? Use the Internet! Entering any term into a search engine (e.g., Google, Ask Jeeves, or Yahoo) can help. In addition, there are a number of glossaries and online computer dictionaries that can help. A popular one is www.webopedia.com, or consult the computer sections available via the Internet Public Library at www.ipl.org or the Librarians's Index to the Internet at http://lii.org.

Performance, 164, 213
  contract negotiations and, 170
  incentives and, 220
  increase in, 97
  standards for, 218, 236
Personal computers (PCs), 26, 27, 210,
  244, 267
Personal digital assistants (PDAs), 28,
  35, 81, 92, 99, 267
Personal health records (PHRs), 6, 8, 91,
  101, 225, 234
  access to, 214
  defined, 5, 267
Personnel resources, checklist for,
  178 (ex.)
P4P. *See* Pay for performance
Pharmacies, 9, 32, 121, 124
Pharmacy benefits management (PBM),
  105, 116, 122, 267
Phase-ins, 72, 209
Phase-outs, 203, 205-7
PHI. *See* Protected health information
PHRs. *See* Personal health records
Physical layout, 135-37
Physician assistants, 240, 244
Physicians' Information and Education
  Resource (PIER), 78, 116
Physician sponsors, 244, 247
Picture archiving and communication
  system (PACS), 127, 267
PIER. *See* Physicians' Information and
  Education Resource
Planning, xiii, xv, xvi, 20, 59, 60, 66,
  99, 110, 138, 168, 175
  contingency, 55-56, 103, 212-13, 257
  cost of, 104, 165
  determining/recording, 119
  flexibility in, 76
  high-level, 148
  implementing, 113, 202, 222
  long-term, 127
  special considerations in, 142-43
  strategic, 240-42
  successful, 73
  team for, 74
  technology, 173
  for training, 194
  treatment, 249
Platforms, 39, 80, 81, 123, 267

PMRI. *See* Patient medical record
  information
PMS. *See* Practice management system
Point and click, 187, 241, 242, 267
Policies, 9, 23, 268
  changes in, 187, 189-90, 237
Portals
  patient, 9-10, 69, 80, 91, 92, 267
  provider, 9, 69, 80, 91, 268
  Web-based, 35, 38, 121
Practice management system (PMS), xiv,
  1, 7, 8, 11, 13, 39, 40, 61-62, 69, 76,
  79, 89, 91, 101, 113, 114, 116, 268
  data in, 207
  developing, 3
  e-prescribing and, 124
  EHR and, 152, 154-55
  implementing, 41, 247-50
  integrated model and, 123
  legacy, 249, 250
  scheduling and, 206
Prescription refills, 69, 116, 138, 192,
  201, 219, 213
  work flow for, 139-40 (ex.), 141 (ex.)
Prescriptions, 9, 62
  electronic transmission of, 79
  formats of, 143
  transactions for, 233
  See also Drugs
Pre-selection phase, 242-44
Printers, 24, 25, 81, 91, 100
  types of, 29, 31
Prior authorization (P.A.), 122
Privacy, 3, 9, 17, 18, 92, 215, 227, 237,
  257, 268
  protecting, xiv, 24, 224
  training in, 249
Privacy and Security Rules, 17, 47,
  48-49 (ex.), 49, 50, 56, 137, 190,
  212, 213, 214, 215, 238, 249
  changing, 201
  implementing, 216
  supporting, 200
Problems, 208
  addressing, 179, 204, 211-12, 220,
  221, 249-50
  insurmountable, 221
Process, 9-10, 23, 148, 241, 268
  changes in, 62, 81, 131, 187, 189-90